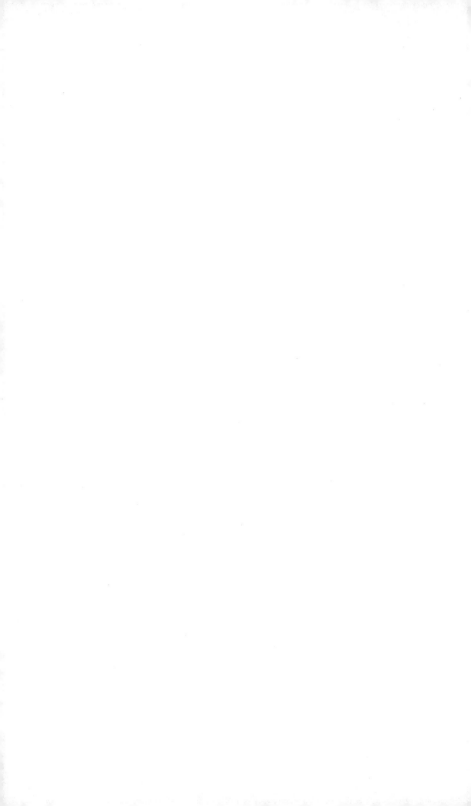

Delivering Effective College
Mental Health Services

Delivering Effective College Mental Health Services

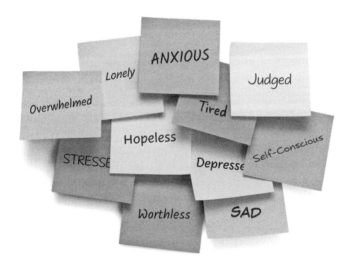

LEE KEYES

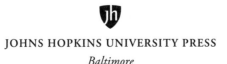

JOHNS HOPKINS UNIVERSITY PRESS

Baltimore

Johns Hopkins University Press
2715 North Charles Street
Baltimore, Maryland 21218-4363
www.press.jhu.edu

Library of Congress Cataloging-in-Publication Data

Names: Keyes, Lee, author.
Title: Delivering effective college mental health services / Lee Keyes.
Description: Baltimore : Johns Hopkins University Press, 2019. | Includes
    bibliographical references and index.
Identifiers: LCCN 2018036805 | ISBN 9781421428857 (hardcover :
    acid-free paper) | ISBN 9781421428864 (electronic) | ISBN 1421428857
    (hardcover : acid-free paper) | ISBN 1421428865 (electronic)
Subjects: LCSH: College students—Mental health services.
Classification: LCC RC451.4.S7 K49 2019 | DDC 616.8900835—dc23
LC record available at https://lccn.loc.gov/2018036805

A catalog record for this book is available from the British Library.

*Special discounts are available for bulk purchases of this book. For more informa-
tion, please contact Special Sales at 410-516-6936 or specialsales@press.jhu.edu.*

Johns Hopkins University Press uses environmentally friendly book materials, including recycled text paper that is composed of at least 30 percent post-
consumer waste, whenever possible.

With gratitude to Lisa, Halley, and Harrison, for their love and support, and to all my family, who taught me to question the prevailing narrative

Contents

Acknowledgments

Heartfelt and special thanks go to Paul Polychronis, David Wallace, and Jon Brunner, for their stimulating conversation and encouragement, and to the many courageous counseling center directors who supported and taught me through the years, often without knowing they were doing so.

I also thank my colleagues and friends at the University of Alabama's Counseling Center and Division of Student Life, who, as partners, worked alongside me as we strove to help students become who they are.

Most important, I am grateful to the students who allowed me into their lives and in so doing taught me how to be a helper. Without them, everything I have ever done professionally would have been impossible.

Delivering Effective College Mental Health Services

Introduction

Mental health is all about problems in living, how one receives them, how one perceives and comprehends them. A mental health delivery system can only be as good as it is accurate in this process, and from the very beginning—actually, even before the very beginning, when clients consume web information and experience the first phone call as they make the often stressful decision to seek help. How these services are structured sets the tone or orientation, which, in turn, may or may not enable the therapeutic work to begin on the best possible footing.

Consider the following three introductions to therapy:

"What brings you in today, Ray?"

"I'm not sure. I'm just 'off,' not really my usual self."

Ray went on to describe feeling apathetic and sluggish, not getting out of his apartment much, watching the world—and his grades—go sliding by. He'd always loved school and had been a fairly cheerful, rambunctious type from the time he was a boy. Ray said these problems began shortly after he arrived at college, and he strained to identify any discrete triggers or negative events. What he did know for sure was that his sleeping was fitful and his usual hungers and thirsts had dried up. What the therapist knew was that his profile for depression was elevated, meaning not good. Ray cried out, "Things can't go on like this."

So what do we think of Ray? Do we file his presentation under clinical depression? A mood disorder? Is Ray overwhelmed or suffering a crisis in confidence occasioned by first failures?

· · ·

"Hey, Angela, what's going on?"

"Who knows. My mom told me I had to come here. I guess because I told her I want to come home."

She elaborated that she had begun to have panic attacks in middle school, and these would come and go for inexplicable reasons. They were back, perhaps a little more frequent and intense now. There were no identifiable or specific anxieties or fears; rather, the episodes seemed unhinged to anything noticeable—*noticeable* being a key word here. Angela was asked how she has been managing the spells, and whether anything made her feel better. "Not really," she said flatly. She sarcastically offered that she would gladly live in a cave if she could, "to get away from everything." Her anxiety had always limited her academic success, which was threatened now because she had been placed on probation. But Angela was indifferent. Now it was her mother's turn to panic.

Perhaps we could diagnose Panic Disorder in this case, since the criteria are satisfied, but we might see this as anxiety masking anger and rebellion, since these had no other safe means of expression.

• • •

"How can I help you, Jacob?"

He bellowed, "This is some bullshit, man. I'm tryna' do my business and I get called names while I'm at it. So, what's a man to do? Say nuttin'? I hit back hard dude, and now they want me to see some old-ass man in an easy chair."

After the initial outburst Jacob allowed only a few morsels of history. An African American, he fought a lot in his predominately white high school. He'd been kicked out of class before and had an arrest or two on his record. Jacob said nothing of his family and wasn't going to. When asked what names he'd been called, he retorted in disbelief, "Whaddaya think?!" There were whiffs of distorted perception and memory, which made the therapist wonder about paranoia. But Jacob was not avoidant or isolated—quite the contrary—and he made decent grades in a tough discipline, engineering. "Let's just get on with this," he would say. "What I gotta do?"

We may see Jacob as belligerent; perhaps he has an underlying paranoid or antisocial character structure. Alternatively, Jacob could be seen as a natural-born fighter, marked with the scars of trauma and righteous indignation.

In these and all other cases, the service and the therapist who represents it have choices to make. In the big picture, therapy openings are brief, say 30 to 45 minutes long, and during this ephemeral time the therapist must offer some magic that is not available elsewhere. That magic is *an accurate and empathic response to all individuals, to their entire history, their entire context, and their possible life trajectory*. This must be achieved quickly, in the first session if possible but certainly by the second. Often, as in the previous examples, the presenting situation is "hot," meaning that someone, somewhere, is wanting things to be fixed, and pronto. The service in which this human theater occurs will have its own requirements, usually involving mundane things like documentation, billing, and triage, that is, choosing the "intervention" path on which to place the client. Some services are flexible in this regard, and some are as rigid and fragile as a glass tube. Some have a narrow focus or lens, while others are broad and expansive. In short, the therapist may be under significant pressure to move quickly and "fit" the client into the perspectives, structures, and pathways provided by the service and facilitated by those who created it—whether the founders knew about that potential outcome or not.

Therein lies the problem. It is possible, when we are not thoughtful or patient, to work with clients in ways that perpetuate their predicaments and are in conflict with the university's mission of learning. How does one avoid that? How can colleges create and implement helping structures that match their mission and the campus culture, and at the same time accurately attend to the full range of their students' needs?

In this book I hope to provide an answer to these and related questions, for both counseling center personnel and the upper administration officials to whom these centers report. As such, portions of the book, particularly the early chapters, are written for those with intermediate or advanced training in college counseling or college mental health, while others provide a basic education for those who have not been deeply exposed to the inner workings and ethics of college mental health. In my view, it is not really possible to propose an organized philosophical or conceptual groundwork for constructing college counseling services without addressing the information needs of practitioners and upper administrators, novices and veterans alike, because it is they who occupy positions in the field. All central features of college counseling services—psychotherapy or counseling processes, outreach services, consultative activity, training activity—will be explored as we discuss the paradigms and models upon which they are based.

A principal orientation of the book is the pursuit of a coherent method of creating an entire college counseling enterprise that is congruent, in all its functions, with the paradigms and service models that best fit its campus culture and student body.

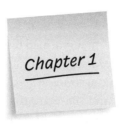

Chapter 1

Mental Health Paradigms and Service Models at Colleges

Though all mental health disciplines can trace their ancient roots to philosophy, it is rare that training programs investigate this very deeply. Graduate students may get a smattering of exposure to philosophical origins in individual class meetings, such as clinical seminars or the history and systems class for psychology, but coverage is often brief and cursory. Even when the topic is broached, one is likeliest to learn about modern views of and approaches to human problems. You hear about Pavlov, Wundt, Piaget, James, Freud, even Pinel, Nightingale, and Dix. This is as it should be, as novices need to know about schools of thought in interventions to advance and improve human welfare.

In some training programs, students may also receive a brief overview of business issues: how to set up a private practice, for example, or discern the ethics of functioning within various agencies, the military, or the departments of state and federal governments. Still, the goal of such conversations is about "functioning within" a model, not so much creating one from the ground up. There may also be some exposure to counseling or psychotherapy paradigms, but these refer to "discrete models or patterns of ideas that constitute theory beyond the therapies of everyday practice. Counseling paradigms, so conceived, represent metatheoretical frameworks for conceptualizing and analyzing the practice of counseling and psychotherapy" (Cottone, 1992, p. 20). These paradigms may be seen as descendants of "scientific paradigms" first outlined by Kuhn (1970). Cottone (1992, 2007) ultimately identified five such paradigms: organic-medical, psychological, systemic-relational, contextual, and social constructivism, and these are the intellectual ancestors of the paradigms I write about in this book. But again, these are organizing metaphilosophies for counseling and psychotherapy specifically, not for the entire construction, enterprise, and science of mental health service provision in any or all of its current settings. They certainly do not speak to the nontherapeutic activities of the modern mental health service: consultation, outreach, and training, or to the business and structuring of all a center's services.

What is glaringly absent from training programs is a deeper study of the philosophy of service orientation and provision: how one goes about selecting the paradigm from which to work and build a mental health service entity; choosing service elements that are consistent with the paradigm; and creating a service model—the nuts and bolts of mission and vision, policy and procedure, programs and services—that flows rationally from these two. Absent, even, is a study of how one might avoid incongruous, conflicting, and even potentially harmful philosophies and metapractices. It seems strange that the field has not addressed this aspect of learning in any coherent or comprehensive manner. Everything a service entity does with clients follows from choices about such things.

The subject areas in the book involve the philosophies and orientations of mental health services in higher education and the decisions that administrators make concerning them. The goal of this book is to give mental health providers and administrators a conceptual basis for structuring these services. Such choices are often made by default or in an unthinking manner, and by individuals who have little or no training in service or business models as they pertain to mental health. This can result in services that do not match local culture or student growth needs. The themes I present include philosophical conflict in service paradigms and how these may be addressed in a rational manner; maximizing theoretical "fit" on campus; identifying influences that may derail service development; and philosophical consistency with student affairs traditions and applied practice. In particular, I highlight a debate concerning the medical, developmental, contextual, and other models, thus posing serious questions about a casual or purely economic integration of such services in various settings. Ultimately, I hope to provide a guide or road map for mental health professionals and higher education administrators who create or amend counseling service structures.

Paradigms

Ask any mental health program student, or even a seasoned practitioner, what paradigm informs the provision of their services and you are likely to receive a blank stare in return. At best they may say something about the "medical model," simply because for many it is the prevailing paradigm, at least in the United States and perhaps other Western countries. But it is not the only choice, even in these cultures. Actually, the medical model is not even a paradigm, in my opinion. It is a service model, as are many other approaches I will outline.

But first, let's start with paradigms. A paradigm is "an outstandingly clear or typical example or *archetype*" (*Merriam-Webster*; emphasis mine). A paradigm is a motif, an original, and as such, it is often copied and repeated. A literature search for paradigms in mental health returns a few items concerning narrower concepts, such as mind-body dualism, technological or neurological approaches to diagnosis and treatment, social determinants of mental health, deinstitutionalization of mental illness, and even one based on risk management. These are all useful concepts, but they lack a sense of spectrum, coherence, and thoroughness in their view of humans.

For the purpose of assuming a philosophical position on how best to deliver services, one needs a more encompassing view of humans and their problems in living, one that is not bound in time, current technology, and culture. Put another way, a paradigm is this "encompassing view," and it includes an orientation toward humans and how one perceives them and their needs. I argue that there are only four paradigms related to philosophy in the structuring of mental health service operations. These are the intrapersonal, extrapersonal, societal, and spiritual-existential (see fig. 1). As applied to mental health, in particular the creation of mental health services, each represents a literal point of view based on the sphere of human functioning one is examining. Deliberately choosing these points will force us to answer questions like: Are you focusing on the inside of the person? How far inside? On the outside? How far outside? The points within spectra are not necessarily mutually exclusive, and in many cases one may blend with or encompass another, but this is only useful if philosophical incongruence is addressed adequately. As Gustave Flaubert said, "There is no 'true.' There are merely ways of perceiving truth" (as cited in Steegmuller, 1982). In the complex task of perceiving and understanding humans and their problems, everything depends on where you are standing and what you are looking at. Let's further examine the four paradigms that encompass the points of view we may choose to assume.

The intrapersonal paradigm. In this motif the location of both human problems and their resolution exists within the person. Of primary interest are patterns of symptoms, disease or disorder, diagnosis, and matching interventions borne out through experience and research. Examples of models based on this paradigm include the medical, health service, psychoanalytic, and, to the degree that physical and emotional growth are of interest, the developmental.

The extrapersonal paradigm. Here the focus is on the full context of the person, his or her total environment. Aspects of context may be seen as psycho-pathogenic, such as abuse, neglect, discrimination, harassment, extreme stress, and poverty. Related

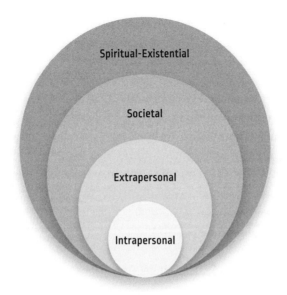

Figure 1. College Mental Health Paradigms

models may include the contextual, ecological or systems, and if life stage and adaptation of the individual are of prime importance, developmental models. Common factors in behavior change, the root of contextual approaches, may be more relevant than treatment-specific factors.

The societal paradigm. In this view, broad societal influences are the target of reduction or elimination of human problems in living. Issues such as social justice, racism, sexism, gender discrimination, inequity in law and policy, and so on, are the focus of both the client's and the practitioner's work. This may be closest to the traditional training and approaches of the social worker and the community psychologist. Most consistent with this paradigm are the human service, public health, ecological or systems, and feminist models of service.

The spiritual-existential paradigm. Spiritual or existential foci are about the place of humans in this world and their transcendence of the harsh realities of life. It involves superordinate goals and the most "cosmic" view of pathology, which may be seen as maladjustment to universal truths. Various faith-based service models and Buddhist or other Eastern practices may be most consistent with this paradigm.

It is evident that these paradigms vary according to "location" or etiology of pathology and methods of resolving problems. They represent a complete spectrum of micro- to macro-levels of symptoms and problems, and possibly well beyond that, to include spiritual or existential matters. Each has its own strengths and limitations, the latter of which may result in incongruous "treatments" and services if one does not take great care in planning and execution. Yet it is possible to proceed thoughtfully and in ways that match the needs in a particular community.

Service Model Definitions

Awareness of philosophically oriented service models is almost nonexistent in the mental health fields. While the notion of a model is well-known in medical health care, in that discipline models focus on the financing of care (Ellwood, 2005; Physicians for a National Health Program, undated). For similar reasons, the concept is often used in business, from which we may borrow a definition. A business model is an "abstract representation of a business, be it conceptual, textual, and/or graphical, of all core interrelated architectural, co-operational, and financial arrangements designed and developed by an organization presently and in the future, as well as all core products and/or services the organization offers, or will offer, based on these arrangements that are needed to achieve its strategic goals and objectives" (Al-Debei, El-Haddadeh, & Avison, 2008).

Models, then, are more about the fundamental aspects of an operation, but these elements, taken together, may or may not reflect the creator's vision, philosophy, or orientation toward understanding humans that are represented in paradigms. A model is the "arms and legs" of the paradigm, which would ideally be reflected in each component of a service, including counseling, outreach programming, consultative work, and training, or would at least not be discordant with it. In keeping with health and business models, Archer and Cooper (1998) outlined campus mental health models, but these centered on types of services offered and intended populations of interest rather than on a guiding philosophy. As the majority of campus mental health services are provided at no-to-very-low cost, the financial and business aspects of a service model are often less relevant in developing the overall orientation of the center. Much more important are the philosophies that guide a predominant view of humans and their problems in living, as that forms the basis of the bulk of work in which such centers engage. While there is some literature pertaining to this topic, most of the knowledge base appears to rest within the professional community itself, in the form of its day-to-day practice and mutual consultative support.

The conceptual grandparent of all campus mental health service models is known as the Cube Model (Morrill, Oetting, & Hurst, 1974). This model described the "dimensions of counselor functioning" in three dimensions, or axes, of a cube. The three dimensions are target of the intervention (from individual to large group), purpose of the intervention (from remediation to development), and method of intervention (from direct service to media). This model was very influential in developing aspirations as to how a center might enhance its offerings in the broadest sense possible. Several of the models I will describe can trace their origins to this model.

In August of 2014 I conducted a brief convenience sample survey of counseling center directors via the listserv of the Association of University and College Counseling Center Directors (AUCCCD). I simply asked them to identify what they considered to be the guiding service model in use at their centers, along with a citation if they could provide one. Of about 700 directors I received a response from 32, admittedly not a representative sample. The purpose, however, was to determine whether anyone at all considered a model to be in use and, if so, which ones might be identified in a cursory survey. The responses I received are divided into categories:

- Biopsychosocial model (actually a subset of the medical model)
- Brief therapy models
  a. Brief intermittent model (Cummings & Sayama, 1995)
  b. Short-term episodic model
  c. Time-attendant model (Burlingame & Fuhriman, 1987)
- Building resiliency and supporting personal success and goals model
- Campus stakeholder model (Jed Foundation, 2018)
- Client-directed, outcome-informed model (Duncan & Miller, 2000)
- Community mental health model
  a. Brief campus-wide services model (Archer & Cooper, 1998)
- Consultation or organizational and community development model
- Contextual/environmental/ecological/systemic models (Wampold & Imel, 2015)
- Cube model (Morrill et al., 1974)
- Developmental model
  a. Broad-based comprehensive student development model
- Educational services model (Archer & Cooper, 1998)
- Feminist model
- Human service model (Hansen, 2007)
- Medical, health service, or clinical model
- Multicultural and cross-cultural models
- Public health model
- Strengths-based model
- Hybrid (of two or more)

In addition to "full" models, two directors identified significant areas of emphasis in their centers: training and evidence-based therapy. Six of the models were purely "home grown," and nine were identified as "hybrids" of two or more models. A few were primarily focused on the psychotherapy function. Among the group were suggestions of more mainstream models, which I have learned about in my interactions with other directors. I will attempt to define these further according to existing literature, scant though it may be. These models include the following, in alphabetical order.

Comprehensive Counseling Center Model (CCC). A recent addition to the debate, the CCC model expands on Archer and Cooper's (1998) concept of the comprehensive counseling services and community development model. This model proposes four pillars of service, including clinical, consultation, outreach, and training functions. The consultative and outreach functions of a center are what define its "comprehensiveness," or its ability to positively impact the entire campus community (Brunner, Wallace, Keyes, & Polychronis, 2017). While a CCC center may choose to focus on a particular paradigm, it is also possible for it to manifest some features of all four paradigms. This is less likely for the other models that follow.

Consultation or Organizational and Community Development Model. As noted by Archer and Cooper (1998), this model focuses on community and organizational improvement through consultations on campus. Direct services with individuals may or may not be emphasized. It is similar to the contextual model in that both are believed to result in enhanced mental health outcomes as a result of their competent and effective responses to the community's needs. What makes it unique, even in Archer and Cooper's formulation, is the potential for individual services not to be among the services offered.

Contextual Model. Here the main factor of interest is a holistic, common-factors approach to student needs, based on common-factors research in psychotherapy (Wampold & Imel, 2015).

Generally, it has been observed that collaboration, empathy, therapeutic alliance, positive regard, genuineness, and therapist factors account for the largest variance in psychotherapy outcome, while specific treatment methods account for very little, often less than 1% (Laska, Gurman, & Wampold, 2014). That is, it is the context of therapy that matters more than specific technique. Extending this view to other aspects of the mental health service, the contextual model seeks to address the entire context of the student, inside and outside the therapy office, in a similar way through consultation and outreach to the campus community.

Developmental Model. This model derives from literature in Student Affairs disciplines as it relates to college student development (Chickering & Reisser, 1993). Of interest are developmental processes in the areas of cognition, psychosocial functioning, identity, morality and ethics, race and ethnicity, sexuality, gender, and more (Garvey, 2014). The goals of counseling centers guided by this model are to recognize developmental stagnation and to work to move students further toward their ideal or maximum development, regardless of their background, presenting status, or mental health condition. A significant objective is improving the likelihood of student success in both personal and academic areas.

Ecological or Systems Models. Based largely on Bowenian concepts in family therapy, the ecological or systems models focus on services for all involved in overlapping circles of human interaction (Lewis, Beavers, Gossett, & Phillips, 1989). Individuals are seen as functioning not in isolation but within larger units, such as families, colleges, departments, programs, roommates and floor mates, friend groups, and other social structures. Each one is seen as conveying emotional importance; therefore, interventions must reflect that reality.

Faith-Based or Eastern Spirituality Models. Models based on faith or Eastern spirituality may be found in religiously affiliated institutions. Principles of faith may be observed not only in therapy but also in consultative and outreach work. However, there are also centers that incorporate Eastern forms of spirituality into their practices with individuals and groups, such as Buddhist and meditative approaches to well-being. Proponents see these models as offering a means to transcend earthly realities through universal principles unfettered by guidelines found in secular work, though the two can be joined in a hybrid model as well.

Feminist or Social Justice Model. Some centers have developed a strong social justice orientation and may also identify as feminist. Social justice may refer to "access to needed information, services, and resources; equality of opportunity; and meaningful participation in decision making for all people" (National Association of Social Workers, 2017). In this model, problems in living may be viewed as the expected outcome of injustice and unequal treatment. Services may be offered to individuals, groups, and other systems, with significant involvement in advocacy and policy development at all levels.

Human Service Model. This model defines counseling in particular as a human service just like law, education, and accounting (Hansen, 2007). In this view, campus mental health services may be defined as wholly separate from health or medical professions and services. These centers may, therefore, focus on any aspects of other models, but not necessarily on such medical precepts as symptoms, disorder, and diagnosis. Professional guidelines and ethics form the foundations on which such services are oriented.

Medical or Health Service Model. In some campus mental health circles, the medical or health service model is referred to as a "clinical" model due to its typically singular focus on direct and individual therapeutic interventions. Predominant foci of interest are symptoms, disorders, diagnosis via the *Diagnostic and Statistical Manual of Mental Disorders* (*DSM-5*; American Psychiatric Association, 2013) or the *International Statistical Classification of Diseases and Related Health Problems* (*ICD-10*; World Health Organization, 1992), and structures that support efficient and billable encounters. The field has also proposed a "biopsychosocial" model, but its main purpose is facilitating a broader understanding of the contributions to disease. Brain-based views of human problems, and therefore medicinal or other physiological interventions, are often of primary interest in this model. Mental health services are often seen as an adjunct to care by a physician, as is the lab, X-ray, or pharmacy.

Public Health Model. This model derives from efforts in violence and substance abuse prevention. It aims "to promote a healthier environment, intensify primary prevention and influence public policies in all sectors so as to address the root causes of environmental and social threats to health" (WHO, 2018). In campus mental health, this model allows for addressing root causes or contributions to mental health burdens by focusing on policy and broad-population-level interventions, while at the same time working with individuals directly.

Matching Services to Local Campus Culture and Needs

An oft-repeated maxim in college counseling circles is "If you've seen one school and center, you've seen one school and center." This refers to the enormous variety in the formulations of campus services in institutions of higher education (IHE, to be used interchangeably with college, school, and university) across the nation and world. Accreditation site reviewers, while hopefully finding adherence to a uniform set of standards—the necessary "skeleton" of a center—also find significant differences in style, structure, service offerings, and orientation of the service. In short, campus mental health or counseling centers mirror the human beings they employ or serve; they have personalities, and these vary. The reasons for this variance are complex, as complex as the college and the community in which the center operates. Essentially, each school is located within a region and a culture, draws its students from dissimilar though sometimes overlapping areas, and has differing demographic profiles of its faculty, staff, students, funding sources, missions, and customs—not to mention the personalities and values of administrators and practitioners. Universities are small worlds, and they are therefore deserving of some right to self-determination and identity, all the way down to every service they offer.

Campus leaders are busy steering a large ship. At the highest levels, they are looking miles and years ahead to not only keep the vessel afloat but also put into the safest, best waters for its passengers. Captains issue orders for all crew to follow based on this information, but they cannot actually offer services directly to them on an hour-to-hour basis. For this, they need manuals and guides and well-trained, responsive crew members. You can find such crew in every department in IHEs, in my opinion—including college counseling centers.

In addition to my 27 years in college mental health, I have worked in hospitals, Veterans Administration centers, service agencies, schools, and private practice. College counseling is unique, as are the other entities. It is a specialty and deserves recognition as such. Every center director can attest that higher education encompasses a broad range of highly nuanced ideas and practices, perhaps more than in most other areas of endeavor. The well-trained staff of a campus service is attuned to those nuances and works with students to interpret and adapt to them so as to achieve both growth and success. This is how we carry out our captain's orders.

There is one big problem, however. Other than accreditation standards, such as those promulgated by the International Association of Counseling Services, Inc. (IACS, the oldest standards set specifically for colleges in the United States), there is no manual—not for service philosophy and orientation or model, that is. Most of the time, administrators and practitioners develop structures and services based on what they learned in their training and read in the margins of current issues and trends, following their intuition and with big hearts. They do an astoundingly good job of this for the most part. Students are served and develop into educated and productive citizens. Sometimes this process is haphazard, a patchwork of building blocks often cemented together in the haste of addressing a real-time fire on board. This is not hard to understand. Life on campus can be frenetic for those serving students. Resources are often limited, so the tendency is to address campus needs quickly, for the sake of customer service, but with too little time and human resources to do it thoughtfully and thoroughly enough. This happens on every campus from time to time and on some campuses often. Some campuses do well in strategic planning, others do not. The best strategic planning is both top-down and bottom-up, and this takes time.

In my travels as a site visitor, I once learned of a college that was working hard and well at formulating its counseling service. In addition to homework they received weeks ahead of time, counselors and administrators had meetings *over a period of three consecutive and full days*. I emphasize this, as I had never heard that before. Even then the planning was not complete. It continued for another six months. This bunch was being thorough, perhaps obsessive—but a good obsessive! In the end the product was a great one; local and professional cultures were understood and respected, and the professionals involved were content. As a result, students were being happily and competently served. This service is thriving.

At the other end of the spectrum are centers with a failure-to-thrive syndrome. In this scenario, no time and little thought are devoted to *meaningful creation that matches needs*. Sometimes the center is thrown together hastily, and sometimes it has existed in a reflexive or unthinkingly organic state for years, even decades. Sometimes its manager was not adequately trained, or was never exposed to college mental health as a field of study and practice, or is a strict adherent to a paradigm or model that does not fit campus needs. Sometimes departments and people are "merged" in a hostile manner, with no attention paid to understanding and respect; only it is not really a merger, which connotes "melding," but more an act of consumption—of meaning, of talent, of possibility, and of hope. These things happen for a variety of reasons, some of which involve a kernel of truth, like personnel problems that have never been addressed directly and assertively, or fierce and pressing financial matters. Occasionally an administrator is persuaded by a charismatic but not altogether altruistic colleague. But, my friends, this is a recipe for failure. Staff members in these circumstances often have serious problems with morale, purpose, and focus. And do not be mistaken: people do not abandon their training, beliefs, and values just because someone has imposed another set on them. In fact, they will tend to dig in further, thus potentially creating long-lasting conflict with the agenda of administrators, no matter how positive in intention it may be. It is better in the long run to take your time and do your homework.

To be fair, mental health professionals can sometimes be viewed negatively on campus, and this too can lead to problematic formulations of services. This view arises in part due to law and ethics pertaining to privacy rights of students, the center's clients. Stakeholders in schools always want more information, usually for good and decent reasons, than is allowable under these codes. This is understandably frustrating, though I have found there are always other ways to address the needs. So there is a professional basis for the frustration, but it is frustration nonetheless. Add to that a posture taken by some practitioners to simply and reflexively say no to such requests for help without offering an alternative, or to fail in supporting the community in other ways through responsive consultation and outreach services, and what you have is an isolated service, the value and purpose of which everyone will question. We can be our own worst enemies at times. When budget time rolls around, it is preferable to be seen as absolutely essential for campus life itself.

Getting back to the topic, How does one orient a philosophy of services in a way that matches local culture and needs?

To do this, one must have reliable data, both quantitative and qualitative, which captures the essence of the community and its people. The information should paint a picture of the people, not only in demographic terms, but also noting their strengths, needs, struggles, and stresses. In gathering this data one must not allow image and marketing, a significant driver of campus practices, to get in the way of facing realities. Every campus, and every community that hosts it, has both strengths and challenges. On many campuses, some groups benefit disproportionately from its gifts while others more often face its challenges. These issues are directly related to the mental health and well-being of the population, and stakeholders must comprehend them if the goal is creation of matching services.

Answering several targeted questions is a good place to start. These questions represent an attempt at understanding both the psychological burden and the degree of support present in a particular community. To the best degree possible, questions should lend themselves to both quantifying and categorizing information, so that planning may more easily follow. Here are some examples of the types of questions that are useful in this stage of planning:

- What is known about the prevalence of diagnosed mental illness, including substance abuse and addiction, in the community? Are some disorders more frequent than others? In whom? What is the state and range of campus and local medical health services? What is the state and range of campus and local counseling and psychotherapy resources? What is the state of health insurance in the area? Do all practitioners understand, respect, and work within one another's professional cultures and values?

- What are the most common physiological stresses for students and others? What is the state of housing, food supply and deserts, clothing needs for the climate, safety, and exposure or vulnerability to crime? What are the most common criminal offenses, and who are the most frequent victims? Where can one go to get help about everything in this list?

- Describe the psychological "ecosystem" of the area. Identify the major components in this system. In what areas might one feel unwelcome or threatened? In what areas might one find affiliation and support? How difficult is it to get there and to gather? How easy or difficult is it to belong?

- What is the prevailing social, religious, and political climate of the area? Who are the privileged? Who are the disenfranchised or marginalized? Who or what is assisting the latter? Does the institution provide or connect to these resources?

- Who works in the intersections of diverse groups? Who are the joiners, and the peacemakers? Who are the dividers, the splitters, the separators? How quickly can the people find or avoid these groups? What is the state of spiritual and ethics resources in the community?

- What opportunities do the people have to increase esteem in self and others? How can they safely explore, create, express, and manifest or actualize their identities and gifts? With whom and where would this happen? Would anything or anyone interfere with these growth processes?

- What key laws, regulations, and policies provide for or constrict the well-being of the people? Is the institution involved in advocating for enhancements or corrections, where appropriate and needed, of these issues?

One could easily fill a book with the answers to these questions—and that is exactly what I recommend you do. This is the homework, the investment, the foundation on which superior services can be built. This is the guidebook for three days of meetings in the act of creation. It is also the inoculation against misdirection and failure to thrive. It is the empirical support for the reasoned choice of paradigm and subsequent service model.

Many things can and have derailed this process. Sometimes it has been an individual, perhaps more than one, who has limited abilities in the area of democratic consensus building. Autocrats and micromanagers are poison to this process, and so are the indolent and indifferent. Beware. But more often, I think much more often, it is unspoken and conflicting agendas that hobble the act of creation. These may be personal agendas in some cases, though serious professional or guild agendas also come into play. Professional agendas may not be altogether unreasonable, having to do with stated mission or the orientation toward the person that a discipline may take. The counseling, social work, psychology, and medical professions all have different points of view, goals, and values, not to mention the codes of ethics and laws that guide them. This is not inherently a negative thing, if one can harness the spectra and variety involved instead of seeing them as a threat.

Guild and economic issues are another matter entirely. With these, power dynamics may appear, and one group may tend toward hierarchy or supremacy over others. (Look carefully at national trade publications, and you will see this clearly.) If the others don't rebel or resist at that moment, you can bet they will later, and it will occur in unseen, uncontrolled ways. This is damaging to the whole enterprise and is often the source of the stagnation and failure to thrive addressed previously. Facilitators must have eagle eyes to monitor for this dynamic, and talons too, for putting a stop to it. Such patterns can also happen with advocacy groups, if they are a part of the process. Some national groups have a strong, if not militaristic, position on mental illness, demanding that resources be devoted only to the most seriously ill. This is wholly understandable given the needs in that population and the woeful state of resources for them in America. Some professionals and advocates will see mental illness in all student behavior, thus overstating the case. It must be remembered, however, that universities serve all students and have the right to define the services they will offer. There is an overarching goal of developing and educating all students, to the best degree possible, regardless of their circumstances. This includes those with mental illness as well as those with other problems in living; both conditions can and do disrupt learning, and both groups should be served.

Creating a Campus Paradigm Map

Once local data has been captured and categorized, you can create a map of paradigmatic themes specific and perhaps unique to a campus. Think of this as a psychological heat map of the community. It helps to assign numerical values to each component of the map, as one might do when matching areas of need with institutional priorities. Or, in another approach, team members can tally what is known concerning various incidents occurring in each area of concern. If possible, this can be done for the answers to all the assessment questions noted earlier. This will of course depend on the availability and accuracy of the data IHEs possess and provide. If data points are missing, time and care ought to be devoted to gathering them. Skipping or giving cursory treatment to this stage can have lasting negative outcomes for the entire process.

Let's work through a few brief hypothetical examples of campus assessments, which are intended to provide a rough overview of what an assessment process can produce. Numbers indicate a consensus ranking of concern.

- A historically black college and university (HBCU), located in a large urban area. This HBCU is respected and politically active in the community, has a history of producing successful leaders, and is closely affiliated with faith traditions. Most of its students are drawn from the immediate area and region. They are disproportionately likely to experience racism and violence in the host community (1). There is campus evidence of issues related to substance abuse among the students (3). Due to funding constraints, this HBCU has minimal supports for academic, health, and counseling needs (2). At the same time, it provides multiple avenues for religious and psychosocial support, as well as mentoring and student gatherings. It has a strong network consisting of local leaders, congregations, and activists. *Suitable paradigms: extrapersonal, societal, spiritual-existential. Suitable service models: faith-based, ecological, social justice, CCC, contextual, public health.*

- A small college located on the outskirts of a town of 15,000. Nearly all of its 1,500 students live in town and commute to class, and the majority will live in this same area or region after graduation. There is little in the way of organic social support on campus. This region is known to have a high prevalence of depression and drug abuse, particularly involving meth and opioids, and relationship violence is frequently reported by local authorities (2). There is one counselor and one nurse providing services on campus, both part time, and local human services are limited (3). Due to stresses in the local economy and the influences noted earlier, academic persistence is of great concern to the administration (1). Leaders are aware of a pressing need to expand informal sources of support in order to create an atmosphere of belonging and "home" on campus. *Suitable paradigms: extrapersonal, societal, some attention to the intrapersonal. Suitable service models: developmental, consultation, ecological, human service, CCC, with attention to creating or enhancing a health service model.*

- A large college in the Northeast, located in a medium-size college town. The school is well-known for its rigorous and competitive academic climate. It has a devoted following, and there are no concerns about attracting applicants; the institution is financially very healthy. There is significant commitment and involvement by families and alumni. It provides both counseling and health services, which are well-staffed and highly respected in those professional communities. Academic and social support opportunities are plentiful. Over the past decade or so, rates of mood disorders, including bipolar disorder, have substantially increased, and along with these, rates of suicide attempts and completions (1). Binge drinking is a significant part of the weekend and game culture and is known to have contributed to the overall mental health burden (3). Reports of sexual assault have recently increased (2). In investigating sources of mental health issues on campus, leaders have become aware of a toxic culture of competitiveness and inhuman pressure to succeed, often defined very narrowly (4). *Suitable paradigms: intrapersonal, extrapersonal. Suitable service models: medical and health service, CCC, developmental, contextual.*

- A medium-size Hispanic-serving two-year school located in the Southwest. Students are largely from the immediate area and region, and a significant number commute and are employed at least part time. Health services are provided by various community resources, and there is an on-campus counseling service, which has an emphasis on career planning and academic success. A significant number of students have had DACA or Dreamer scholarships and face hurdles due to their undocumented status, including recent raids by ICE, which have resulted in detention and deportation (1). Heavily utilized support systems include churches and extended family networks (2). In the last decade, there has been a documented increase in issues related to substance abuse and relationship violence (3). In spite of these and other challenges, the school is well-known for its contribution to the arts and humanities. *Suitable paradigms: spiritual-existential, societal, extrapersonal. Suitable service models: social justice, faith-based, ecological, CCC, contextual.*

• A large NCAA Division I institution located in the Southeast. Well-known for its athletics and Greek life programs, this school has a large and reliable following across the nation and is financially stable. Students come from every state, with a significant number from other nations. Nearly 60% identify as female. The institution has steadily raised its academic standards, and many students from regions with less academic preparedness report a high degree of related stress (2). Thought to be partly associated with this stress is a high prevalence of substance abuse and addiction disorders, as well as sexual assault and rape (1). Growing diversity among the student population has resulted in some tension within a politically conservative climate in the region, including bias incidents (3). This university has many supportive resources available, including extensive health and counseling services. *Suitable paradigms: extrapersonal, societal. Suitable service models: developmental, contextual, CCC, social justice.*

Special Considerations for Developmental and Contextual Views of Students

College students have a great many needs across many dimensions of experience, including the academic, spiritual, relational, psychological and emotional, physical health, financial, occupational, and avocational spheres of college life. Each of these dimensions, were we able to graph them on paper, would appear very different in scale, orientation, and overlap for each student, and yet each student needs access to various forms of support and learning in all of these areas if we are truly to fulfill our mission of retaining and producing ethical and contributing civic leaders.

An individual's life dimension profile places him or her in a specific context. No student lives and functions in a developmental or an ecological/contextual vacuum. It is true that each student brings his or her own internal or biochemical endowment, but one cannot fully understand the total student without placing the student in context.

Mental health service entities have choices to make concerning which service model they will follow. The most basic choice relates to the medical model, which is based in content-derived symptoms and diseases, and the developmental or contextual models, which are based in process-derived states of growth transitions and management of stressors in context (Hayes, Villatte, Levin, & Hildebrandt, 2011). Each model begets related choices concerning funding priorities and goals that are rationally linked to different units of interest or focus. In the medical model, the unit of interest is the student's symptom or disorder, which must be treated and alleviated. In developmental or contextual models, the unit of interest is the student's growth pattern, which is either enhanced or limited by their total context.

As an illustration, consider a student who has been diagnosed with ADHD (Attention-Deficit Hyperactivity Disorder) or Bipolar Disorder. Each diagnosis requires meeting the criteria of a specific list of symptoms and symptom clusters. Suppose you meet such a student and you find he or she is also experiencing one or more of the following contextual factors:

- Stress related to global political and marketplace influences
- Extremely poor sleep routines and hygiene
- Arrhythmic lifestyles or, more simply put, chaos
- Too much screen time, not enough play and exercise
- A paucity of trusting, mutually satisfactory relationships, in any sphere
- Racism and discrimination
- Increased sense of threat and diminished opportunity for affiliation

- Poverty, or resources insufficient to being a good student
- Alcohol and drug abuse
- Poor nutrition
- The inherent transitional "volatility" of the late adolescent and young adult
- The seasonal and cyclical nature of stresses in the academic environment
- Violence, rape, sexual assault, harassment
- Environmental toxins in the food supply or living environment

It is not uncommon to meet students managing half or more of these factors, yet these may be discounted in purely medical orientations. If we were able to somehow bathe students' brains in these factors, what would those persons look like? How would they be likely to behave? Might they have problems with attention? Or disruptions of energy?

Benefits of the Thoughtful Orientation of Counseling Services

Orienting the focus and philosophy of a campus counseling service need not be, nor should it be, an unthinking activity, or an activity of convenience, economics, or politics. Ideally, it will be purposeful and embedded in the deepest traditions of promoting the education and success of the greatest possible majority of young adults. Typically, these traditions are most consistent with a range of theory that undergirds Student Affairs divisions (Garvey, 2014). After all, *all* students experience developmental and contextual challenges. Students experience homesickness, roommate or family conflict, stress from academic demands, communication difficulties, peer pressure, cultural biases, identity confusion or misdirection, and so on, at very high rates. The prevalence of specific medical/psychiatric diagnoses among college students ranges from, say, 2%–5% of the general population. It makes sense, then, to orient campus counseling services accordingly. It is known that allocating resources toward the lower and middle quartiles of a distribution results in greater degrees of problem mitigation and prevention.

Orienting counseling services toward a student's overall development also provides for the greatest reach into the various cells of the classic cube model of counselor functioning (Morrill et al., 1974), including each type of target, each purpose of intervention, and each method of intervention. In a purely medical model, the focus of interest tends to be on the remediation of the individual's condition at the level of direct service alone, and the role of campus consultation services is deemphasized and many times nonexistent (Brunner, Wallace, Reymann, Sellers, & McCabe, 2014). This results in allocating resources to the sickest, who are much farther along in the development of chronic health problems, and there is a place in the world for this. The point is not whether one model should predominate; it is that there should be room for a wide range of approaches to the broadest segment of the campus population possible. I argue that IHEs obtain the optimal cost effectiveness and problem mitigation when each point in the spectrum of human life problems can be addressed.

Breadth and Depth of Developmental or Contextual Models

Professionals providing services in developmentally and contextually oriented counseling centers provide human services and not health services per se (Hansen, 2007). This means that a college counselor is free to address any human or life issue a student may bring, even those that may fall outside the scope of traditional diagnostic tools. This model confers advantages to students in concrete, observable ways. One does not have to be "sick" to go to counseling in such centers, because no concern or issue is too small or too large to discuss with a counselor. This results in a better probability of seeing students much earlier in the cycle of problem development. It also allows for an entire course of counseling to be focused on acquiring skills that are needed for future success, such as assertive communication and healthy coping behavior. In this sense, the college counselor is also an educator and may advocate for the student outside the counseling hour, or engage in activities other than traditional "clinical interventions." Furthermore, such centers are firmly focused on learning that will last a lifetime. Not insignificantly, the increased comfort in accessing such positively oriented services also results in a greater likelihood that students will reach out to this service in a time of more intense crisis.

Traditional-aged college students are living through a psychologically volatile period. They pass through various stages of identity and skill development, some of which are painful (Chickering & Reisser, 1993). This results in rather intense reactions and behaviors that, while perhaps unsettling for all involved, are essentially transient—unless, perhaps, something occurs to arrest the student's development. One week a student may appear very ill; at another time he or she appears calm and coherent. It is easy to mistake transient but intense mood states for serious illness, thus running the risk of pathologizing normal, albeit occasionally alarming, behavior in some settings. Developmentally oriented centers are primed to "tolerate" intensity, firm in the knowledge that the psychic stew will settle down for most students. Holding this intensity in a safe environment allows the student to pass through it unscathed, without acquiring potentially lifelong labels and, most worrisome, a damaging and limiting conception of self as "sick"; and yet it also allows for the learning that needs to take place. Counseling provided from this point of view places a priority on having adequate time with the student, in order to accurately determine her or his full context and needs. The amount of time required for this is typically not available in medical facilities.

Applicability of the CCC Model

CCC personnel work diligently to orient the center's mission and services to serve the greatest number of students in need. This is done with much forethought, research, and exploration based on local experience, which is preferable for the orientation of any center (Brunner et al., 2014). All four aspects of the CCC mission (counseling, outreach, consultation, and training) may incorporate a developmental and contextual philosophy that seeks to meet students where they are, develop the strengths and genuine identities they possess, encourage them and give them hope and confidence, and address their life problems at the same time. Without care and nurturing, these approaches can become disjointed and misaligned with the student's growth needs.

When such centers are acquired by a medically oriented entity and folded into their operations with little thought and planning, some predictable losses or reductions of function occur. These include both perceived and real privacy; outreach; prevention; consultation; mental health screening; groups; programming; well-developed relationships with the administration, faculty, staff, and community professionals; community and campus liaisons; functionally coordinated teams; strategic directions aligned with those of the university and student-learning outcomes; services proven to positively influence retention, graduation, and academic performance in positive ways; networking and exchanging information with other higher education professionals; immediate phone consultation; training residence hall staff; assigned committee participation; consulting with students concerned about another student; staff trained in young adult development and strength-based counseling; and simply a more warm and supportive environment.

In my work with IACS, I have seen firsthand that such centers may lose their accreditation status due to thoughtless mergers. In reality, these mergers are more like acquisitions in which the counseling service is consumed whole by the host; little to no actual integration is attempted. Generally, these losses occur when the counseling service is viewed primarily as a resource for those providing medical services, much as a pharmacy, a lab, or an X-ray department does. This posture results in the failure-to-thrive syndrome in the counseling service and should, in my opinion, be avoided; the many benefits of other models are worthy of continuation and support. Therefore it is my recommendation that centers remain independent and autonomous, though accountable to campus partners, in the pursuit of the mission. Models of interdependence can also work well, provided there is intentionality in joining cultures and philosophies.

CCC Goals and Needs

The CCC works continuously to refine its developmental and contextual philosophy and orientation toward students and its campus community. It views students as functioning within a developmental trajectory and an ecological context. The goal is to meet students where they are functioning in this matrix and assist them by advancing their development to the next stages, while at the same time mitigating and resolving crises that may limit their successful growth and academic success. In this sense, the work is driven by a client-centered and directed focus on their developmental needs. CCC proponents believe strongly that students must have a resource that allows them to experience life crises, contains the negative effects of same, and facilitates a passage through them to a maturity as whole and enhanced as possible. They believe that many life problems arise from poor contextual adjustment and alignment and that a conception of self as ill is neither necessary nor ideal for most students. These dynamics are reflected in the fact that rates of mental illness are not increasing, although rates of student distress continue to rise (see Chapter 2). This strongly indicates that student adjustment and coping-skill repertoires should be of primary interest on campus. CCC advocates also believe strongly that adequate time must be devoted to these ends, which is why weekly counseling sessions last 50 minutes as opposed to 7- to 15-minute encounters every month or two in other settings.

The CCC also views members of the campus community as essential partners in addressing the overall well-being of students. In this work, personnel consider the whole campus environment in all its aspects as part of student context and ecology. It considers its staff, who are licensed by the state, to be a panel of educators and experts who work in close, interactive collaboration with students and various constituencies to support positive, strength-based approaches to emotional health, as well as prevention and early intervention in student life problems. Staff members are seen as student advocates with a broad range of case management skills. This important part of functioning on campus is apparent in direct services as well as consultative, outreach, and training activities. Many services, such as crisis intervention, are available around the clock and calendar and are not otherwise available to students. CCC services are also convenient and inexpensive, without the longer term impact associated with third-party billing. The CCC is a resource that seeks to incorporate soft skills, such as social and emotional learning, emotional intelligence, and ethical awareness, into the student learning experience. These skills are known to be associated with positive emotional well-being and academic success. Top-tier counseling services maintain these services while addressing direct student need through good rates of utilization.

In Chapter 2, I examine data concerning the needs of college students, which should further inform campuses concerning the broad orientation of their services to match those needs.

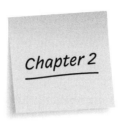

Chapter 2

Developing an Accurate Picture
of College Students

College students are arguably the most studied population in the West. From surveys by various organizations and industries, to Psychology 101 research participation, information about them abounds. In fact, there is so much information it can be difficult to get a clear picture or determine what is relevant. Media reports are even more confounding and, in my opinion, often misleading. Consider the following headlines.

- "Are College Students Getting Sicker?" (psychologytoday.com, December 29, 2010)
- "An Open Letter to All the Fragile College Students in Their Safe Spaces" (townhall.com, November 14, 2015)
- "Why Are Millennials So Fragile?" (mindingthecampus.org, January 2, 2017)
- "College Students Need Remedial Classes in How to Be Adults" (thedailybeast.com, September 1, 2016)
- "In the Wake of a Suicide Epidemic, Inaction Speaks Louder Than Words" (psychcentral.com, May 23, 2014)
- "The College Student Mental Health Crisis" (psychology today.com, along with a rebuttal titled "Why I Don't Believe Reports of a Mental Health Crisis," February 15, 2014)

Pretty dismal stuff. It has become commonplace for some to use language like *epidemic* when discussing the mental health of college students. But, as a noun, this term refers to the widespread occurrence of disease. As you will see, there is in fact an epidemic, but it is of dis-ease, not disease.

The Epidemiology of Emotional Well-Being in Students

What does epidemiology have to say about college student mental health? First, let's examine data for the general population in the world and in North America. In a global study, Merikangas, Nakamura, and Kessler (2009) state:

> A recent comprehensive review of the field of child psychiatric epidemiology noted that the number of observations in community surveys of children and adolescents has risen from 10,000 in studies published between 1980 and 1993 to nearly 40,000 from 21 studies published between 1993 and 2002. The results of these studies indicate that about one out of every three to four youths is estimated to meet lifetime criteria for a Diagnostic and Statistical Manual of Mental Disorders (DSM) mental disorder. *However, only a small proportion of these youth actually have sufficiently severe distress or impairment to warrant intervention.* About one out of every ten youths is estimated to meet the Substance Abuse and Mental Health Services Administration (SAMHSA) criteria for a Serious Emotional Disturbance (SRD), defined as a mental health problem that has a drastic impact on a child's ability to function socially, academically, and emotionally. (emphasis mine)

Merikangas et al. (2009) go on to say that about one-fourth of youth experienced a mental disorder in the past year, and about one-third do so in their lifetime. Census data tell us there are about 42 million youth in the United States, about 13% of the total population. This would translate to about 11 million youth with any kind of mental health burden in the past year. For the 20 million or more college students in the United States, that number would be about five million. It is not known what "small proportion" of this number actually warrants intervention, though that can be surmised from other data presented next.

It should be noted here that the authors also rightly point out problematic issues related to definitions and methodologies in such studies across the globe. Furthermore, at this writing, the United States is the only nation in the world still relying on the *DSM-5* for diagnostic purposes, as opposed to the *International Classification of Diseases* (*ICD-10*), published by the World Health Organization (WHO, 1992) —although the *ICD-10* is now being more broadly implemented here.

The National College Health Assessment (ACHA), 2016, revealed that 7.6% of students—about 1.5 million—reported having had a psychiatric condition of some kind. This falls below the one-quarter estimate cited earlier, but is perhaps within the range of those actually needing intervention. Also in the United States specifically, for those over the age of 18, the age-adjusted average prevalence for serious psychological distress in the past 30 days is 3.5%, or a little more than 11 million people (Centers for Disease Control and Prevention, 2015, table 46). For those 18 to 24 years old, that figure is 2.5%; for all women, 3.9%; and for all persons of color, from 1.9% to 4.5%. Most tellingly, for those below the poverty line, it is 9.1%. As you can see, context is everything. For suicide, the prevalence rate for those 15 to 24 years old is 11.5 per 100,000 (CDC, 2015, table 17). For college students, the same estimate is 7.0 per 100,000 (Schwartz, 2011). In what may be the most precise reporting on this topic, from the United Kingdom, the rate for college students is 4.7 per 100,000 (*BBC News*, June 25, 2018). If you are in college, you are actually buffered from the outcome of suicide compared to your same-age peers.

What are the trends in the prevalence of mental health issues and disorders? As there is no single, uniform repository of related information, this is even more difficult to determine, but there are some relevant data and other clues. Looking again at the CDC's report (2015, table 46) on the age-adjusted average prevalence for serious psychological distress in the past 30 days, this time for those aged 18 to 24, the population proportions for six time periods are as follows:

- 1997–1998: 2.7%
- 1999–2000: 2.2%
- 2001–2002: 2.8%
- 2004–2005: 2.5%
- 2010–2011: 2.4%
- 2013–2014: 2.5%

These data clearly indicate stability over a 27-year period; notably, nothing resembling an epidemic. In Canada, it has been reported that about 4.8% of its population experiences depression annually, and this prevalence diminishes with age (Patten et al., 2006). In another CDC report (2015, table 30), the prevalence rates for suicide among those aged 15 to 24 is presented, this time per 100,000 and over a longer time period:

- 1950: 4.5
- 1960: 5.2
- 1970: 8.8
- 1980: 12.3
- 1990: 13.2
- 2000: 10.2
- 2010: 10.5
- 2013: 11.1
- 2014: 11.5

These data indicate a significant increase between 1970 and 1990, followed by a slight decrease and leveling in the decades thereafter. The increase took place in the years after the Vietnam War, Watergate, and four separate economic recessions in the United States—significant stressors in that part of its history. It is often reported that suicide is the second or third leading cause of death among college students (Eiser, 2011), and media reports have used the term *epidemic* for this cause of death, but again the data actually reveal a decrease since 1990 and stability in prevalence since then. Data for years after 2014 should show us what has become of these rates since then. In addition, the CDC data is for all 15- to 24-year-olds, and given the findings by Schwartz, one can extrapolate that the data for college students is likely to be significantly lower.

Recently, the CDC released an additional report on U.S. suicide rates (CDC VitalSigns: Suicide, June 2018). It reported that suicide rates increased in nearly every state between 1999 and 2016, with an increase of 30% or more in half of the states. But it added that 54% of people who died by suicide did not have a known mental health condition. Due to a multiplicity of contributory factors identified in their data, CDC principal deputy director Anne Schuchat later stated that "suicide is more than a mental health issue" (*CBS News*, June 7, 2018). These factors included "relationship problems, substance abuse, physical health problems, job- or money-related stress, and legal or housing problems," which mirror findings from other data sources, discussed later.

In his landmark study on the mental health continuum, represented by the concepts of languishing and flourishing, Keyes (2002) notes the following:

> A diagnosis of the presence of mental health, described as flourishing, and the absence of mental health, characterized as languishing, is applied to data from the 1995 Midlife in the United States study of adults between the ages of 25 and 74 (n = 3,032). Findings revealed that 17.2 percent fit the criteria for flourishing, 56.6 percent were moderately mentally healthy, 12.1 percent of adults fit the criteria for languishing, and 14.1 percent fit the criteria for DSM-III-R major depressive episode (12-month), of which 9.4 percent were not languishing and 4.7 percent were also languishing.

Though the population here is generally older than the traditional college student, and the source data is now dated, the languishing are a clear minority of the sample, and the majority of those with a history of a depressive episode were not languishing either. Keyes's mental health continuum is easily applied to college student life—indeed, to all campus life—and will be discussed further.

Center for Collegiate Mental Health Data

There are many interesting and relevant data points in a recent Annual Report of the Center for Collegiate Mental Health (CCMH), 2016. This report noted the following: "The 2016 Annual Report summarizes data contributed to CCMH during the 2015–2016 academic year, closing on June 30, 2016. De-identified data were contributed by 139 college and university counseling centers, describing 150,483 unique college students seeking mental health treatment (a 50% increase over last year); 3,419 clinicians; and over 1,034,510 appointments" (p. 1). Given that all participating centers are using identical instrumentation, the data are among the most robust gathered concerning college students and their mental health. Regarding trend data, the following is noted:

- Lifetime prevalence rates of "threat-to-self" characteristics (nonsuicidal self-injury and serious suicidal ideation) increased for the sixth year in a row (p. 5). This persistent trend, combined with dramatic increases in demand for mental health services documented in the 2016 report, confirm that counseling centers are evaluating and managing increasing numbers of students who may also represent "threat-to-self."

- Despite increasing demand marked by risk, lifetime prevalence rates for prior mental health treatment remain stable for the sixth year in a row (p. 4). One in two students who sought treatment had had counseling, one in three had taken medications, and one in ten had been hospitalized. The six-year stability of these trends suggests that students referred for counseling do not have increasing rates of pre-existing mental health concerns.

- Anxiety and depression continue to be the most common presenting concerns for college students as identified by counseling center staff (p. 9). In addition, students' self-reported distress levels for depression, generalized anxiety, and social anxiety continue to show slight but persistent increases each year for the past six years (p. 6). Other areas of self-reported distress (academics, eating concerns, hostility, substance abuse, and family distress) have remained relatively flat or are decreasing.

• Thus, not only are anxiety and depression the most common concerns, but students' distress in these areas appears to be growing slowly, while other areas of distress are flat or decreasing. These findings highlight the fact that not all aspects of mental health are worsening and that it will be important to better understand the role of depression and anxiety in college students. It seems clear that rates of distress are high and slowly climbing and that students are accessing assistance at higher rates than is indicated in national prevalence data. The question is why.

The lifetime prevalence rate data for mental illness are consistent with what has been reported in epidemiological studies in both America and Canada, as noted. It strongly suggests that the cause of the increasing rates of "threat-to-self" are not due to rates of preexisting mental health issues. These data run counter to what is often stated in the media and by some industries or vendors. Taken together, all of this suggests that other factors are at work in terms of self-harm, there is no "epidemic" in college student mental health, and millennials are not "sicker." What is true is that students are distressed and are using services in ever-increasing numbers, which to me is an indication that awareness is increasing and outreach efforts are working. I believe that extrapersonal and societal factors are involved in rates of distress, including developmental trajectories and contextual stresses of the highest order. Also relevant are the coping-skills repertoires of today's students. One cannot assess stress without also knowing about how students adjust to it, or not.

Threat to self or self-harm, broadly defined, is the turning inward of distress. Key questions are (1) what is causing the increase in this distress if it is not preexisting mental health concerns, and (2) why are students focusing inwardly in manifesting their distress? Clues are available in the "list of top concerns" data from the same CCMH report (p. 10). First, suicidality is ranked 18th of 44 items by counselors choosing the top concern, whereas self-injurious thoughts or behavior is 24th. Thus, while these appear to be increasing, they are *not* anywhere near the top-most concerns, suggesting that actual risk is low and that counselors believe other concerns need more attention. Looking at those top 24 rankings, we find that 14 of them have an external or environmental influence, such as stress, family, trauma, or relationship problems. Stress is ranked number three among all items.

The Role of Stress in Modern Life

A hypothesis, one born of the extrapersonal and societal paradigms, is that modern life is becoming *intolerably psychologically stressful*. It has been noted widely that previous generations faced dire circumstances and death and got through this with resilience and grit. There is no doubt that, at least for many, we have more resources and conveniences than ever. But that is not really the point. Today's youth do not have a clear path or ritual into independence and adulthood, and they are struggling to define what success, which seems so easily attainable by others, means for them. The world is an increasingly confusing and frightening place. What we are seeing are reactions to an extreme form of impotence and frustration among our youth, and I think many arrive on campus ill-equipped to cope. Further, the caring adults in their lives are overwhelmed by the effort to prepare and equip them for these challenges.

Before exploring this subject further, it is important to look again at information claiming or suggesting the existence of mental health epidemics. Data from such sources are often cited in media reports, with attention-getting headlines like those noted previously. This occurs even when the entity producing the data has the best of intentions in responding to the needs of students. Any mental health professional can promptly testify to the frustrations involved in interviews with the media. Nonetheless, apparently alarming information fuels the presses. For example, until recently an oft-cited data point—"73.1% of college counseling directors believe they are seeing increased severity of concerns in students"—appeared annually after directors were surveyed (American University and College Counseling Center Directors, 2015). For years this figure hovered around 70% to 90%. Many outlets made it a focus of alarmist articles. What readers could not know is that directors could only choose "increased," "decreased," or "unsure" in response to that item. "Stayed the same" was not an option until 2016. When that response choice was included, the results were 57.1% increased, 23.8% stayed the same, 0.8% decreased, and 10.8% unsure (AUCCCD, 2016). To be sure, 57.1% is still of concern. In this figure I believe directors are expressing concern about managing both the increased demand for services and increased prevalence of self-harm ideation and behavior. In other words, it is a rational concern. But others, for a variety of reasons, conflate the data with the occurrence of mental illness or just plain "sicker" students.

In 2012, the National Alliance for Mental Illness (NAMI) conducted survey research on 765 college students diagnosed with a mental health condition and who were either currently enrolled or had been within the previous five years (NAMI, 2012). In addition, only 37% of the respondents were of traditional college age, well below the overall proportion in enrollment. In terms of mental health issues, 51% had a mood disorder diagnosis (depression or bipolar disorder), while 11% had an anxiety disorder diagnosis. Six percent had a diagnosis of schizophrenia, and 1% had a diagnosis of a substance abuse–related disorder.

It would be a mistake to conclude that "over half" of students have a mood disorder, but I heard that said by advocates with my own ears. It would also be an error to conclude that only 11% of students have issues with anxiety or that 1% have substance abuse concerns. A glance at the CCMH data shows us that the prevalence of such concerns is much higher—concerns, not necessarily diagnoses.

Similarly, a web resource for the Jed Foundation, a national nonprofit advocating for college student well-being, starts out with an appropriate title: "Students with mental troubles on rise; Colleges add suicide response teams, counselors" (Jed Foundation, 2017). But on the same page the following language is used: "Other colleges in the state [New Jersey] also are seeing more students with mental illnesses. The increases mirror national trends." Here, in a single resource, we see the conflation of distress with mental illness. This tendency is a reflection of the intrapersonal paradigm at work. It is a form of cognitive bias derived from the paradigm, which can occur in all paradigms. This is not to say that distress and mental illness do not overlap; they clearly do. But extrapersonal, societal, and spiritual-existential factors are also intimately involved—likely more so, in my opinion.

Returning to survey data from ACHA, a casual reader is not likely to see that 7.6% of college students have a psychiatric condition of some kind. They are far likelier to read that, at any level, 58.5% felt hopeless, 75.5% felt very sad, or 40.5% felt so depressed it was difficult to function, in the last 12 months (ACHA, 2006). Incidentally, these figures have remained stable in the annual fall data taken since 2000. The key word here is *felt*. This is again a reflection of the level of distress reported by college students. Media and industry representatives widely reported that 40% of students are *depressed*, having keyed in on that word, and translated the data into "depression," not felt experience. In a subsequent publication you can see the subtle conflation of terms:

Though our survey was not primarily focused on mental health care provision, this component of the care of college students has come to the forefront of discussions about health and safety on many campuses. National trends in mental health needs on college campuses have gained significant attention in the last several years. The 2007 National College Health Assessment data reveals that 43.2% of 20,500 student respondents on 39 college campuses felt "so depressed that it was difficult to function" at least once in the 12 months prior to taking the survey. Data from the "Healthy Minds" study from the University of Michigan shows that 17% of respondents screened positive for depression at the time of the survey administrations in 2007 and 2009. While these statistics place college students at about the same risk of mental illness as their non-college attending age counterparts the need for mental health care on campuses is substantial and some data regarding mental health service will be included in this analysis. (ACHA, 2010)

The reader will note the reference to screening for depression. The use of depression and other mental health screening instruments has become commonplace in higher education, most notably through the resources available at Screening for Mental Health (2018) and Healthy Minds, as noted previously. However, there is evidence that such screening activities involve problems with high false positive rates (identified as often above 50%), and some organizations have actually recommended against their use outside of programs of formal assessment and treatment (Thombs et al., 2012). Thombs et al. further elaborate that the effect size for screening on actual occurrence of depression "is virtually zero." Such instruments may be capturing the mood state of students when they are in the midst of a moment, albeit transient, of emotional volatility. Such states occur frequently among late adolescents and young adults, especially in the college environment, which poses many novel and challenging stresses for them. But these pass as the student adapts and learns to cope, which also often happens rapidly. This pattern may explain why high false positives for screening occur for college students.

There is, then, a distinction to be made: subjective distress, no matter how high it may be, is not necessarily equivalent to or indicative of mental illness. It is the subjectivity on which we need to focus in order to discern all of the factors contributing to the felt experience of distress. It is critical that we move beyond targeted, binary questions found in surveys, the results of which are based only on self-reports. Proximal causes of phenomena are relevant, but so are broad, distal influences—more so as one focuses beyond well-trodden intrapersonal factors. Extrapersonal, societal, and spiritual-existential paradigms lend themselves to the investigation of more remote, more nuanced, and perhaps more deeply influential contributions to distress. These paradigms produce the following questions.

- When not indicative of true mental illness, what do high rates of distress suggest about stress and coping in youth?
- What societal or cultural pressures are involved in the generation of both stress and coping?
- Within the dynamics listed here, what role is played by families and educators in the preparation of students to manage distress?
- What is known about an institution's local patterns of distress in students?
- How well is the campus prepared to assist students in learning to negotiate intense but transient mood and stress issues?

These and other questions will be addressed in the next chapter. The general tone of media, industry, and advocacy group reports is that the deficits of interest exist within students—again, an intrapersonal paradigm perspective. Let us suppose, however, that these deficits may actually exist elsewhere, in other groups or organizations of people, in societies, in nations, and in the world. Let us imagine that what we are seeing is the outcome of young people attempting to adapt to these issues, in many cases entirely on their own—which is to say, with little competent direction or guidance from supportive others. Lest the reader think this is an example of parent-blaming, let us further propose that older adults are also struggling to manage larger-world contributions to distress. Evidence exists to support these notions.

In the American Psychological Association's Stress in America survey (2017), results indicated a shift from earlier sources of stress. For the first time since 2006, political climate and elections were identified as a somewhat or significant source of stress, with 57% endorsing the contribution of the current political climate, 66% the future of our nation, and 49% the outcome of the election as causative. The effect was most prominent in urban areas. Significant concern for personal safety rose from 27% in 2009 to 34% in 2017. Concern for police violence toward minorities rose in every major ethnic group. The most recent survey showed a significant increase in stress for the first time in its history. The most cited factors adding to stress were the economy, mass shootings and gun violence, and terrorism. (As an undergraduate in the 1970s, none of these factors was even remotely in my consciousness.) Thirty-nine percent of respondents said their ability to manage stress has remained the same, suggesting that skill development may not be keeping up with newer or more intense stressors.

What are younger generations saying about stress? From the APA report:

> Similar to recent years, in the August survey, younger Americans (Millennials and Gen Xers) report higher average stress levels (5.6 Millennials, 5.4 Gen Xers, 4.1 Boomers and 2.7 Matures) and are more likely to say their stress has increased in the past year compared with Boomers and Matures

(38 percent of Millennials, 36 percent of Gen Xers, 25 percent of Boomers and 18 percent of Matures).

Millennials are also worried about police violence toward minorities (49 percent of Millennials, 29 percent of Gen Xers, 33 percent of Boomers and 22 percent of Matures say this is a very or somewhat significant source of stress for them). A greater share of Millennials also think this will be a very or somewhat significant source of stress in the next few years (49 percent of Millennials, 34 percent of Gen Xers, 35 percent of Boomers and 24 percent of Matures).

Overall, Millennials, Gen Xers and Boomers are more likely to say they engage in stress management techniques (88 percent of Millennials, 93 percent of Gen Xers and 88 percent of Boomers compared to 78 percent of Matures). However, Millennials and Gen Xers are more likely to say they do not feel they are doing enough to manage their stress (30 percent of Millennials, 25 percent of Gen Xers, 13 percent of Boomers and 5 percent of Matures).

The younger generation reports higher levels of stress than older adults and also reports feeling less capable of managing it. It may be this pattern that exaggerated popular news story titles are actually referencing. All forms of stress, including that which arises from home, work, and trauma, are believed to contribute significantly to the overall "disease" burden, which has been called a "modern day hidden epidemic" (Kalia, 2002). Kalia estimates that stress-related disorders alone cost the United States $42 billion annually. The role of stress in the well-being of college students was further underscored in the most recent director's survey by AUCCCD (2017). For the first time, stress ranked second among the most frequent concerns of college students, at 39.1%, topped only by anxiety at 48.2%. (I believe one could question how both therapists and students are defining anxiety, and to what degree it is distinguishable from acute stress reactions.) Depression fell to third place, at 34.5%.

The World Health Organization recently identified nine areas that are deemed broad social determinants of health (2018). If we exclude those involved in health care delivery itself, these areas are employment conditions, social exclusion, women and gender equity, early child development, globalization (including "trade liberalization, integration of production of goods, consumption and lifestyle patterns, household level income"), and urbanization (including "stimulation of job creation, land tenure and land use policy, transportation, sustainable urban development, social protection, settlement policies and strategies, community empowerment, vulnerability reduction and better security"). These areas vary widely among human populations and are thought to capture an enormous amount of variance in health conditions and health-care outcomes across the globe. These are, in fact, the contexts in which people live, and by definition they cannot be addressed within the intrapersonal paradigm alone.

Examining a relatively recent part of modern life, social media consumption starting after 2010, Twenge, Joiner, Rogers, and Martin (2017) presented strong evidence of a relationship between "screen time" and adolescent (13- to 18-year-olds) mental health, particularly among females. They state:

> Depressive symptoms, suicide-related outcomes, and suicide deaths among adolescents all rose during the 2010s. These increases follow a period when mental health issues were declining or stable (see Table 1). Between 2009/2010 and 2015, 33% more adolescents exhibited high levels of depressive symptoms (item mean of 3 or over; 16.13% in 2010, 21.48% in 2015), 12% more reported at least one suicide-related outcome (31.93% in 2009, 35.80% in 2015; 5% more since 2011, 34.21%), and 31% more died by suicide (5.38 per 100,000 population in 2010, 7.04 in 2015).

The reverse is also true, according to this study. Those who spent more time in other social and physical activities experienced fewer mental health issues after 2010. In this view, a young person's social context may be a powerful determinant of his or her emotional well-being. Given what is known about the role of relationships in the developing adolescent brain, this should not come as a surprise to anyone (Siegel, 2014).

In a prior study by Twenge (2000), a massive factor analysis focused on rates of anxiety over a 40-year period, the author concludes that the average person in the 1980s had a higher rate of anxiety than the average psychiatric inpatient of the 1950s. Clearly, the increase is "real." However, Twenge believes that the increase is primarily due to two factors, both of which are environmental or ecological: an increased sense of danger or threat in the world and diminished rates of affiliation with supportive others. These remarks mirror the patterns in data already cited.

Interpreting the Data

Paradigms influence both data production and its interpretation. This is especially true when the paradigm has become associated with an industry, as exists in the medicine-pharmaceutical-insurance system triumvirate. When this association forms, it constitutes a significant source of bias in research and publication, which may overwhelm a reader or front-line service provider, and this bias is even more intense in the consumption of popular media. It takes precious time to dig deeper and understand how forces outside the person are affecting what occurs within him or her. Yet the data are there, waiting for discovery and interpretation. The intrapersonal paradigm is best suited for working with dynamics that *solely or predominantly* originate from within. This is extremely valuable because we will all face problems originating from within, in the form of disease process, sooner or later. It does not, and in my opinion cannot, effectively take into account extrapersonal, societal, and spiritual-existential factors, perhaps because there is no easy way to bill insurance carriers for serving those needs. While forces outside the person affect all of us, nowhere is this more relevant and acute than in the emerging adult, if only because of their lack of experience and, for those in college, their distance from the familiar and from sources of support.

It is like a perfect storm. At this particular time in history, recent generations in America are conscious of a multiplicity of choices, more than their parents had, certainly many more than their grandparents had, which, paradoxically, creates anxiety and stress of its own: pressure to do the right or best thing (Schwartz, 2003). College students are also facing societal and global stress, just like the rest of us, but while mainly on their own for the first time, and after many have been either under- or over-cared for, resulting in poor preparation for adequate coping. Crucially, all this is happening while students are being offered the most convenient, most comprehensive, and least expensive assistance they will likely ever have in their lives, through the myriad programs, services, and relationships that an IHE provides. While we older adults chafe and moan over these stresses and resort to various forms of good and bad coping, the young adult acutely senses the impending doom that "adulthood" seems to offer parents and families. But they find themselves in a community *where it is now possible* to manifest the strain and receive the needed attention for it.

Why, in heaven's name, would we be shocked when they act accordingly? Why would we assume that it is they who are sick?

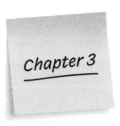

Developmental and Societal Factors Fueling the Clinical Picture

In this and subsequent chapters, I examine themes that may be well known by mental health professionals but are often less familiar to higher education administrators. The latter group may include deans of students, assistant and associate vice presidents, vice presidents, and various personnel in the provost's and chancellor's offices. Although there are exceptions, for the most part these professionals do not possess degrees in the mental health professions or developmental psychology, but they may have been exposed to student development theory, which historically has been commonplace in higher education administration programs.

Even so, there are also many practitioners entering college counseling who may not have been deeply exposed to this same material, and who did not complete an internship in an accredited college counseling service. The material presented henceforth is intended for them as well. The objective here is not to condescend; it is rather to not assume that all practitioners and administrators possess a similar fund of information. In my experience, that has not been the case. This dynamic may be partly responsible for uninformed choices regarding college mental health.

What Is the Full Context of College Student Behavior?

Evidence is plentiful that, for many, modern life is difficult. Surveys on stress, such as those provided by the American Psychological Association, repeatedly demonstrate high levels of stress in the United States and other nations. Of course, earlier generations also experienced stress, which some characterize as even greater in its intensity. A casual review of that history reveals higher rates of mortality from many causes, fewer conveniences and comforts, more technologically primitive forms of health care, and in some cases, a greater sense of impending threat (as that posed by Nazi Germany and the Axis powers). There is something, however, that set such threats apart from those in modern life: clarity. It was less difficult in those times to determine who or what was out to get us.

Today our stresses are much more complex. Information now travels quickly, almost instantaneously, and is obsolete within hours. Global political and marketplace dynamics reverberate through nations and cultures, causing rapid shifts in relations, law, and military preparedness. We are confronted by the stark reality of jihadist, non-jihadist, and domestic terrorism on a daily basis, and in frequent shocking breaking news segments. Impending doom is still with us, but now it seems it could come from anywhere and at a moment's notice.

The landscape in higher education has also endured seismic shifts as state legislatures have reduced funding due to shrinking budgets and regressive practices. The pool of high school graduates has also shrunk, as the baby boom and its echo have faded. Fierce competition for that pool is now a part of every president's multifactorial headache. Leaders and consumers are questioning the value of a college degree, and efforts to grade institutions and their products are afoot. Millennial and later generations are also doing some serious soul searching and are creating novel pathways to adulthood and independence—some of which do not involve higher education. Parents have headaches of their own as "boomerang" students return home, often with no discernible plan for the future. With the advent of decriminalization of marijuana, a distinct drug culture, which preaches taking the path of least resistance, has emerged. For some, this path may involve avoiding the school-to-degree-to-fixed-career transition into adulthood, which they see as the "failed" pathway taken by previous generations.

This drug culture has a point. Youth have witnessed the stress and frenetic pace of their parents, their apparent sadness or meaninglessness when they come home after a workday spent slaying dragons. They also see the hypocrisy in the "adult" world; chaotic and dysfunctional relationships (often one result of intolerable stress), various forms of discrimination in spite of apparent religious beliefs, and a general sense of mean-spiritedness as the world adapts or fails to adapt to "others" in flight from oppression. Many have decided they want none of it, even if it means being uneducated and poor. They are keenly aware that their parents' earning power is less than half what it was for their grandparents, and signs say this may worsen as economies shake and sputter, or even fail altogether.

On the other end of the spectrum are those who somehow believe they should start out, after graduation, earning a six-figure salary—or feel pressured to do so, either by family or MTV's *Real World*. After all, social and other media make it seem as though such glamour is easily attainable, or ought to be. If your Snapchat story is not as attractive as Brittney's down the hall, there is something wrong with *you*. Family members are aware of the contrasts involved and fret over how to help their children measure up and get into the right sports, the right pageants, the right parties, the right organizations, and the right schools. The energy behind this imperative is so keen that parents often take it upon themselves to navigate the systems themselves, giving birth to the archetype of the "helicopter parent" (Glass & Tabatsky, 2014). The psychological origin of this energy is a fear of failure, or, even deeper, a fear that "I am not good enough myself."

Developmental Considerations in the Experience of College Stress

Before we look more closely at the role of parenting in college, we must ponder the interaction of student stress and developmental processes in the late adolescent and early adult. Late adolescents and young adults need space and time to develop an authentic self. While there are of course a great many contexts in which this can occur, perhaps few are better suited to the purpose than the higher-education environment. In my view, when carried out well, this opportunity is a major benefit of the college experience.

During such a time, youth are exposed to ideas, knowledge, experiences, social feedback, and a wide range of relationships that either enhance or detract from personal growth and fulfillment of latent promise. A forming adult can benefit immensely from this environment, which represents an incubator of the emerging self. In this way students experiment, explore, and try on various selves to see which one fits and works the best.

It is both an exciting and a trying time, for students as well as those around them, especially loved ones. The experimentation brings highs and lows, successes and failures, flashes of brilliance and the pain of mistakes. But these ups and downs are absolutely necessary, assuming we all want to produce healthy, competent, and productive adults. Older adults, be they professors, administrators, family members, or friends, simply must respect the need for this period of incubation. Sheltering young adults from all pains can harm them significantly, though we should of course protect them from the most serious ones if we are able to do so. There were times in human history when there was no such thing as this kind of incubation, due to the hardships many faced, but we can, and should, provide it now.

Respect requires allowing enough space and time for growth to occur. For parents this means gritting one's teeth and teaching what one knows, but allowing students to venture off, even when mistakes are a near certainty. Doing this, a sense of faith and trust is communicated, which is the fuel on which the emerging self thrives. It means patience in the face of a tattoo, purple hair, exploring a major that is a "bad choice," financial incompetence, or partnering that causes heartburn. The incubation can take a long time, but learning does occur. Students learn on their own what will and won't sustain them in life, because life itself teaches them. We parents don't always have to do the teaching, as much as we want to. Attempting to do that, we actually interfere with natural consequences and learning, slowing down and disrupting the process of development.

Parents and administrators alike should give youth space and time to incubate the self, and trust that the self will unfold in the way it should, one way or another. Students should take the opportunity to learn about and become who they are. Just as they have the freedom to do so, so do they have the responsibility to accept the feedback they will receive, and to adjust accordingly.

Not that there isn't a debate about these dynamics. Not long ago, the president of a college in Oklahoma penned a note on the school's website in response to a student who apparently complained about feeling victimized by a sermon there (Piper, 2017). Piper pointed out rather adamantly that higher education is for learning, which often involves, by definition, sometimes feeling uncomfortable. He expressed the same frustrations felt by many in the field who struggle daily with the unreasonable expectations of students and others. As higher education has adopted business models, it has also acquired a customer service orientation—not that this is always a bad thing. It can be good to improve one's services and meet customers' needs. Sometimes, however, this progresses into an orientation of entitlement, such that the customer may demand the product (a degree) with as little discomfort (dissonance or struggling) as possible, much as one might do when one purchases, say, a pair of shoes. This obviously flies in the face of traditions in education since the time of Socrates. Further, those of us in the mental health professions know that any growth worth achieving is difficult, while the rewards of the struggle are enormous and life altering.

In another part of the blogosphere, a student countered with her own message that the notion of the coddled college student is a myth (Sampath, 2017). Sampath rightly points out that a great many students have real struggles overcoming trauma, discrimination, and harassment. She notes that today's students may be more vocal in their search for recognition and equality in education. There is truth in this, though I believe more so for the individual; group activism on many campuses is at an all-time low.

The two authors are each right, even though they capture trends in education from different vantage points. This should not be surprising, since one is an administrator and one is a student—populations that often do not see eye to eye. We should listen carefully to both. Incorporating and adjusting to the student experience is paramount if we hope to remain relevant and just in our work. At the same time, we need to uphold reasonable boundaries with respect to expectations or else we diminish our product, an educated and balanced citizen, substantially. Should we understand who our students are and how they best succeed? Absolutely. Should we allow their parents to schedule appointments for them or lobby for a better grade? Positively not. As with most things in life, the truth is somewhere in between. We should work to find it. Ultimately, if college is to be a successful incubator of self, it must apply *heat*.

Mindfulness of Expectations

Mental health issues are best viewed in their entire context. Claims of increasing mental illness among our youth are overwrought, in large part because they fail to consider context. One important aspect of context involves the expectations of students, as well as of those around them.

As already noted, learning and growth are supposed to be uncomfortable. Refining one's approach to thought and decision-making is a difficult business, as we must separate bias from rationality and objectivity, the dross and gold of education. Costa (2016) sees this as a process of unlearning, to which recent cohorts of students are reacting poorly as a result of their expectations for their college experience. In particular, she sees this as a clash between the inherent stresses of learning and a mindset that overvalues performance ratings, preconceived notions of success, discomfort with ambivalence and doubt, and a hyper focus on outcome rather than process.

This view deserves more consideration. It could help explain, for example, high rates of self-reported distress in the absence of true or moderate to severe mental illness. It is consistent with observations concerning modern parenting practices, the coping skills repertoire of adolescents and young adults, and data that support rapid positive changes in these dynamics with just a modicum of support or counseling (Center for Collegiate Mental Health, 2017). In the popular press we often see polarizing comments about higher education, parents, and students, and this is not useful. It is the interaction of all three, mediated by the expectations of each, that deserves our attention, investigation, and application to higher education practices.

From her family, primarily her mother, Kerry learned that college was a time to develop connections in order to improve, or at least maintain, her lot in life. This included new friendships and friend groups or organizations, but it also clearly involved further cementing old family ties and the business affiliations among them. It was not an insignificant imperative to attract and marry the right partner by the time she left college. Her dalliances were tolerated, within the restrictions of her social stratum, as long as she did not truly care for or invest in these partners.

Kerry arrived on campus and immediately commenced the work on these social objectives, and at first was not in the least disappointed. She was bright and energetic, and beyond the initial academic adjustment, classes were not difficult for her; nor were they on her immediate psychic radar. She thoroughly enjoyed the ready-made social schedule her student organizations afforded her, which more often than not included other children from the old families back at home, some of whom she'd known since early childhood. Her reports of the first months in school were met with approval, even celebration, by her family, long before any actual grades had been earned. She even received a call from a state legislator who sang the praises of the affiliations she was constructing. "This is going be very good for your future, Kerry. I see great things ahead for you." How can one not feel confident after a call like that? But she did wonder how he knew about what she was up to.

After her first year, and after a rare quiet time at home for the summer, Kerry had a chance to decompress from all the social noise and partying. She was happy to get a break from trite, adolescent conflicts among her friends. Late in the spring a bout of infighting had broken out in one of her groups and, though she had initially participated in it, she grew weary of it and now just wanted to be away from it. Her sleep had become fitful and restless, not in small part due to the bacchanalian revelry she was expected to join in several nights per week. Kerry had never been a worrier, but now she found herself ruminating over embarrassing and frustrating situations with friends. Her confidence began to give way under a growing awareness that her promised and glorious "future" was not truly free and came with certain strings attached. In addition to establishing and maintaining connections, the conditions also seemed to include drunken carousing, sexual assignations, and, paradoxically, maintaining status and image. "I feel like I've gone to summer camp and can't go home," Kerry thought to herself. Increasingly, she felt as though she was living in two worlds, and neither one was of her own making. Still, and even while at home, she felt compelled to stay up to date with texts and social media notifications, which she responded to at all hours of the night. Her friends' story lines and photos seemed more fun and glamorous, even now, while all she felt like doing was sleep. She wondered if she was one of the losers that her friends talked about. Late in the summer, her mother prodded her to get motivated, to "get back into the game," as she liked to say.

Which she did. Everything resumed as it was before, but Kerry found herself making small escapes, trying not to be noticed. During her first year, she had made other friends of whom she did not speak much. Some were from other parts of the world. One was an instructor who challenged her to find her own voice, as he detected in her writing a lack of authenticity, a parroting of commonly heard social themes. In his class there was brief coverage of feminist values to which she had never been exposed. She had an epiphany that her education was lacking, in both past and present. Kerry was curious as she had never been before. She hungered for expanded horizons but also felt obligated, though trapped, by the social contract with family and friends. She was more anxious and irritable now, and her friends made backhanded comments about her "not being herself," of being more withdrawn. "We didn't see you Thursday night," they would say, with a vague but noticeable disdain. Sensing dissatisfaction among her friends and family, Kerry turned to one defense that had always worked, at least for a short time: avoidance. She began isolating herself, sleeping during the day, and skipping classes for the first time in her life. A friend had given her Xanax at a party once and promised more to boot. Kerry wasn't too fond of it at the time, but now she found the calming, even dulling feeling to be helpful. She took it often now. Formerly full of energy, she was now sluggish and aloof. Her grades began slipping.

At home for a holiday, she was confronted by her mother and grandmother. They knew about her grades and the Xanax. They also knew, somehow, about Victor, from Venezuela, with whom she had been spotted in the student union. Kerry erupted in rage, something she had never in her life done, especially with the family matriarchs. She screamed about the stress they were causing her, that they were responsible for her grades. She stormed off to her room and slammed the door. Later, her mother contacted their minister, a school administrator, even the legislator, to ask them to "talk some sense into her." They tried, each in his or her own way. But it did not work. It could not work.

Kerry "had" symptoms. You could call it depression. Or anxiety. Or substance abuse. Or perhaps one of several other "conditions." But none of these captures the essence of her predicament. She was caught in the clash between expectations and the inevitable search for genuine self that all healthy young adults must pursue. This pursuit cannot be stopped, as the self is always seeking manifestation, but it can certainly be derailed or co-opted by well-intentioned loved ones and even by the school if it does not have clear boundaries about such things. A great many cases of failure to thrive involve, at their core, a self derailed by a host of expectations from many people, including students themselves. It is frightfully easy to contribute to this predicament; all it takes is a lack of awareness of the impact of expectations, their relevance to students, and the realities of development in young adults. When this lack of awareness becomes institutionalized in some way, the IHE will unwittingly defeat its own purpose.

The Necessity of Failure

Some view Western culture, and American culture in particular, as one that places a premium on the success and advancement of the individual. Critics of this view argue that this premium diminishes some individuals and groups, but others say that this does not necessarily have to occur, that one can promote the interests of the individual and society at the same time. (See the works of Ruth Benedict and John Kenneth Galbraith for references on that subject.) In my experience, it takes an educated and enlightened individual to pursue "success" and also orient that success to higher purposes, such as benefiting larger and larger circles of human beings.

Enter typical college students and their families. As noted earlier, they tend to arrive being very focused on pragmatic issues, such as living arrangements and choice of major. There is a tremendous amount of energy devoted to moving the late adolescent and young adult along a continuum of advancement, however that may be conceived in family ethics and values. Getting good grades, joining the "right" organizations, and networking for future employment are, in the minds of those involved, locked in rather tightly. Variance from this template is often frowned upon, if not met with punitive consequences.

College life is, however, a crucible for the formation of both individuality and responsibility, or conscience. Mistakes and failures are inevitable and are the stuff that catalyzes the higher calling of the young adult. In his book *How Children Succeed*, Paul Tough (2013) theorizes that noncognitive skills such as persistence, resilience, and fortitude are actually the bases of future success, though it is cognitive skills that often get the attention. In this view, mistakes and failures are desirable, the launching pad for growth. In short, one gets intimately acquainted with one's self, with both talents and foibles, through a cycle of failure and growth.

Such is the process of learning who we are, what we can do, and the limitations presented by our perceptions and biases. The process of "advancement" is much more earthy and sobering than Western mythologies would have us believe. It is very much two steps forward, one backward, a thousand blind alleys to ten workable paths. This process is to be embraced, not belittled. Great achievers like Newton, Edison, Curie, Einstein, and Carver all said so. Families can be wonderful allies in the young adult's search for self by understanding this failure-and-growth cycle, by welcoming it, and by patiently waiting for their children to learn life's lessons. Students will succeed in their journey to selfhood by minimizing anxieties about social perfection, or, better yet, rooting them out altogether. It takes courage to advance. Fear won't get us there.

It has been observed that, without proper guidance, this cycle may overwhelm and consume students. Mental health issues may arise from a great many sources in higher education. An important source is the situation in which we find ourselves, or our total context, in particular as it interacts with a current developmental stage of life.

Students often find themselves in novel circumstances, something they have never faced before, especially when they are challenged or stressed. Major life transitions are certainly like this: our first serious relationship, marriage, employment, having children, the loss of loved ones. And college! College is itself an extended period of incubation and growth, full of excitement and many challenges. Depending on our developmental history, we are all in different stages of readiness for this enterprise.

Ideally, we will be prepared, at least in some rudimentary fashion, through having had experiences that approximate the transition. Families can certainly provide these, and many do. It is also true that many do not. It is further true that, sometimes, there may be nothing that can prepare us for the stresses we face, whether in college or elsewhere. That's just the way life can be at times.

Imagine that you find yourself in an overwhelmingly stressful transition. You may learn to adapt, gaining the skills you need to adjust and succeed. You may do this through trial-and-error learning, or you may deliberately catch it early and seek more efficient forms of learning, maybe by visiting your campus counseling center or obtaining other forms of assistance. Or worse, you may founder. There is some evidence at both the undergraduate and graduate levels that many students experience a gradual disintegration in functioning and subsequently take a break or withdraw altogether (Patterson, 2016). For some, this disintegration may be due to an underlying mental illness that had not fully emerged before the stress. For others, actually the majority, the symptoms reflect a lack of preparedness, which can be remedied by focused short-term interventions in therapy and other support. Data from the center in which I work indicates fairly rapid equilibrium and restoration in functioning after, say, five or so therapy sessions, which supports the latter conclusion. This pattern can be seen on a regular basis in campus counseling services, but one rarely hears about it.

The difference between the two patterns is critical. This is one reason that accessing campus counseling services is so crucial, especially in the early stages of a stressful transition. Such services can determine what type of intervention is best suited for the emerging difficulties, limit negative outcomes, and increase the probability of continued success.

There are some common themes among those who stagnate. With the help of a film of the same name, the phrase *failure to launch* has entered the common lexicon—not that it needed that help. Many a college parent has experience with the issue, whether it be direct or a vicarious source of chronic fretting. Once, on a flight home from our nation's capital, I even overheard a prominent legislator musing over his student's launching issues. It was difficult to avoid thinking that we are beyond hope if such a well-connected student was having a problem with developmental stagnation. But of course no one is beyond hope of successful transition into adulthood.

There are many factors involved in the maturation process, many more than can be addressed here, but I have noticed a few recurring themes among students struggling with emergence into independence. In no particular order, these are:

- Lack of information or inadequate education. Some students have just not been exposed, for whatever reason, to the world of employment and career making. This group does not know where or how to begin. A solution: Go to the career center and learn what is known about career success.

- Privilege and entitlement. There are some students for whom the words *no*, *limits*, or *deference* are unfamiliar. This group often demonstrates adaptation deficits in the areas of ambition, diligence, labor, and "paying one's dues." They may also feel unchallenged and bored. A solution: Go to the counseling center and work on adjusting expectations.

- Lack of resources. Many students have the knowledge and the willpower but not the financial or other necessities for taking the next steps in advancement. This one is harder to address, but not impossible with enough persistent creativity. A solution: Go to financial aid and pursue the labyrinthine network of scholarship and grant funding.

- Aiming too low. Students sometimes drift downward in their selection of friends, activities, and goals. It's tempting and easy to do the thing that's, well, easy. A solution: Find a mentor and be mindful in your choice of heroes.

- Too much partying. It bears repeating that excessive partying can dull the senses and result in loss of motivation for enjoying the normal vicissitudes of living, like the rhythms of sleeping and waking, resting and working, pleasure and discomfort. A solution: Go to the counseling center and stop numbing out on life.

As already mentioned, there are other contributors to this problem, but these are some big ones. Parents have a role in monitoring these dynamics long before their children arrive at college. It is ideal for rich dialog to begin in elementary school, if not earlier. Even small children have opportunities to address the themes at various developmental milestones, such as first attending school, first exposures to some form of labor and service to others, first responsibilities to others or pets, first earning of income, and so on. Too often we parents let these pass by, assuming the lessons will be learned and achievements earned. Those young adults who remain frozen in stagnation will tell you this assumption is faulty indeed.

It is also possible to overdo it. Visionary Steve Jobs was once interviewed on PBS for its "One Last Thing" documentary (Public Broadcasting System, 2011). Speaking about insights that resulted in his life's work, he said:

> When you grow up you tend to get told the world is the way it is and your life is just to live your life inside the world. Try not to bash into the walls too much. Try to have a nice family life, have fun, save a little money. That's a very limited life. Life can be much broader once you discover one simple fact, and that is—everything around you that you call life, was made up by people that were no smarter than you. And you can change it, you can influence it, you can build your own things that other people can use.

These are profound words, and not just for building things. They describe key aspects for identity development and processes that limit it. In my work and personal life, I am too often struck by how much judgment we humans seem to deliver—to ourselves, to others, to ideas, to thought, to dreams. I and those with whom I work encounter it daily, and many times a day. In my middle age I have come to ignore most of it, but this defense was hard won and took too long for me to develop.

Among other things, college mental health professionals work to help younger adults to spot judgments that inhibit the genuine trajectory of the self. There is no growth without risk-taking, without "bashing into the walls" on occasion. We must all learn to manage unnecessary and harmful inhibition in order to become who we have always been.

There is certainly a place in life for social feedback, for learning from others what we are and are not doing well or effectively. But we ought to critically examine all feedback and determine for ourselves what is "true" and healthy for us and the world around us. This takes time and practice, and the earlier one starts the better. It is not easy figuring out where the world's great institutions of family, ethics or faith, school and government have gone astray. Certainly each has something to offer, to help us reduce chaos and create meaning. Institutions are made of people, so there will not be perfection in these pursuits. It is up to us to sort that out.

Sooner or later, everything that comes to us in life will be categorized as "belonging to me" or "not belonging to me." We simply cannot accept all reflections of us as though we were carrying a mirror around with us at all times. Attempting this will overwhelm the self and lead to poor mental health outcomes. We have to be able to turn the mirror around and perceive that judgment is often more about the other or a system that is in need of our gifts and talents. We don't always have to live "inside the world," but we do have the responsibility of changing that world for ourselves, and for others, if we are to be authentic selves.

Ben was lucky in his small-town high school. His family was well known and popular, and so was he. His parents had both been athletes in their youth, and Ben received a good measure of this gift, which he displayed on the baseball diamond. His team went to the state finals each year of his high school career and won it all his junior year. Aside from a minor injury one season, his athletic pathway occurred in a straight, escalating line of one success after another, from T-ball through minor league recruitment. During all that time Ben had never experienced a losing season or any waiting on the sidelines, except for that brief stint on the disabled list. He dated a lot and pretty much called the shots in that arena as well. Ben created a long wake of broken hearts behind him. Some considered him a grade-A jerk, but in his universe, this had the same effect as zero.

He was smart enough, that is to say, he possessed sufficient analytical cognitive abilities to make school easy. He missed a lot of classes and could still pass exams with a B or better, though his girlfriends or others whom he would hit up for help would gladly do so for a little payback somewhere along the line. Ben was a smart-ass in school, and everyone just seemed to let it slide. He told sexist and racist jokes, which were met with giggling by those who could not, by virtue of their fortunate histories, feel their sting. The decorations on his monster truck included spotlights for field parties, a big "Ain't Skeered" sticker, and a Confederate flag. He had other stickers on his rear bumper, but it—and they—didn't survive a mud-riding escapade. It lay in a creek somewhere, he reckoned. Once, during a baseball tournament on the coast, Ben and others got caught drinking beer on the beach and spent a few hours in the local jail, but his coach and home county sheriff, both acquaintances of the police chief, were able to spring them loose. Ben didn't even know how this happened. His coach wanted him to focus on the game. Ben was a lucky guy. Except none of it was luck, and whatever you want to call it, it was about to change.

Ben was playing in a showcase scrimmage hosted by a big state university when his career came to an abrupt end. He'd hit a long ball in the gap and tore down the base paths with great fury, rounding second and trying to beat the throw to third. The ball, Ben, and the third baseman all met at the same time just ahead of the bag, and right at the foot of the fielder. Ben's knee buckled at the stop, and he felt two enormous pops, which were loud enough for the front row to hear. At first he did not comprehend what the physicians were telling him and his parents. He'd rarely heard a no before; it was always a "No, but . . . ," or a "Yes." So the finality of it all took all summer to register. He rehabbed, and it was coming along well with the help of painkillers and not a little boozing and female attentions. Autumn was coming, and he knew he would at least keep part of his big state school dream alive by attending and continuing his life's party there, lost and depressed though he was.

At first he didn't know what to do with his time, which seemed to be plentiful compared to his practice and game schedule in high school. But he hung out with a group of high school friends who had gone to the same school, and they continued in the activities begun there. He missed a lot of classes, same as before, but still got by, though with much lower grades. At mid-terms, Ben committed three violations during a single event, which brought him before the conduct office. First, he was cited along with others for alcohol violations during an impromptu party in one of the residence halls where his then-girlfriend lived. At that same party, Ben drunkenly attempted coercive sexual contact with another female student, who later also filed a complaint. A passerby noted a Confederate flag hanging in the window of the party room and reported it to the campus police. The flag belonged to Ben, though he claimed that he had not hung it there.

As a result, his girlfriend left him, having seen the party photos on Snapchat, and Ben found himself before the conduct board. He was confounded by this seemingly sudden cloud over his life, as he was no different than before. He asked his father and former coach to come with him to the hearing, but only his father was permitted. Ben was found responsible in some measure for all three violations and was assigned the requisite educational and community service consequences. He was also referred to the counseling center to be evaluated and possibly work further on his obvious ethical shortcomings. Even now, Ben was still lucky in that he had escaped formal assault charges, only because the victim just wanted him to leave her alone and put the whole episode behind her. By the Thanksgiving break, Ben was in the hottest water he'd ever felt. His parents were furious over his grades, and the school he'd always dreamed about was keeping him on a short leash. He entered the spring with an academic suspension looming—a total suspension if he committed one more infraction.

So began his therapy, and ultimately his transformation. Ben's therapist was seasoned and firm with him about his lapses in morality and judgment. Ben was cavalier and surly at first, attempting jokes and ridiculous debates about civil rights and freedom that fell on the ears of a wise elder and went nowhere. For one of his sanctions, Ben spent time with underserved, largely minority children in town. He developed a sort of kinship bond with one boy, superficial at first, as Ben, for the first time in his life, felt downtrodden himself. Once, while delivering items to the boy's home along with his supervisor, Ben witnessed white men in the neighborhood hurling racial slurs and other derogatory words at the limping boy while he played basketball in the street. Ben felt anger and almost came to blows with the men, until his supervisor counseled restraint. "He has to live here, you don't. Don't you give him another problem to handle after you leave." He later told his therapist that he had never considered things from that perspective, and it made him wonder what else he had missed. "I feel like I've been asleep my whole life."

It took more than a full year, but Ben began turning things around. He grew. He had experienced a wall in his life, a wall of failure and pain. Life itself was telling him that his path was not viable and that he must change. Within the failure were seeds of growth sown by those who cared enough to plant them, by setting boundaries and showing him another way. The school itself provided the mechanisms for this to occur, in keeping with its mission of developing students, of moving them along in the arc toward their ideal selves. And all this occurred in the context of the young self in the community that needed and expected more from students.

The Role of Parenting

The college context, along with the sometimes volatile developmental processes of its youngest members, produces a psychic stew through which students must navigate in order to grow.

What in heaven's name is a parent to do? How does one prepare a child for this cauldron of stress? It seems like an enormous task—not just for parents and families, but for administrators as well.

Well, the task *is* enormous. Parents and others must have wisdom, patience, tolerance, and faith to help produce an authentic, productive, and healthy adult. These traits combine not only to weather crises but also to *see them as a gift*. Again, the college years can be a volatile time for students. Late adolescents and young adults are caught between two worlds—that of their youth, their homes and families, and that of their future, their developing selves and careers. This time is marked by both great excitement and great anxiety, which is a recipe for emotional turmoil and crisis. The excitement derives from a sense of increased freedom of choice and independence, as well as the invigorating challenges and risks this brings. To students, the world can seem like a grand buffet, and they are made dizzy with all the delicious offerings. They set about sampling the world to see what it is like, what appeals to them, what fits them, and what does not. This sampling often frightens others, notably parents, but it needn't. Most students figure out on their own what works well and what does not, because the world will let them know. If one gorges on the buffet, pain will be felt.

There is also anxiety. Increased freedom is often noticed by the student very early on, and there is much joy and revelry attending this realization. Soon thereafter, sometimes very soon, a sense of responsibility emerges, which can be quite shocking and as heavy as a coat of lead. It becomes clearer, because life itself will reveal it, that students ultimately cannot avoid being responsible for themselves, for their identities and choices, for the well-being of their friends and communities. For some, this journey is slow and painstaking; for others, it is as quick and awesome as lightning.

It is in this cauldron that emotional or psychological crises occur. At times the friction between these two forces becomes more than the student can bear, much like two tectonic plates colliding. Something has to give. The crisis is the equivalent of an earthquake, the means by which equilibrium is achieved and a new topography is born. For many who interact with students, there can be a strong urge to dampen down the crisis, to soothe the eruption of emotion, to medicate away the discomforts, to relieve them of the responsibility to self and others. While some students may need such interventions, because of the degree of their impairment, many, if not most, do not. In short, the crisis needs to occur, and if we prevent or distort it we are doing students and their future authentic selves a great disservice. Growth does not occur without some pains, and sometimes the pains are quite intense and dramatic.

We therefore find ourselves in a predicament of our own. Using wisdom, good judgment, and the best advice, we have to choose when and how to support the student. We have to balance the need to soothe against the student's need to develop into a mature being. This is admittedly not always an easy task. Tragedies, which have occurred across the nation, have resulted in an attitude or climate of fear for some, and this can produce defensive responding when great patience and faith are needed instead. Unfortunately, the litigious among us, lawyers, and even the courts can unwittingly reinforce this harmful posture through the apparent expectation of clairvoyance. Growth occurs in the process of getting through the pain, not by going around it.

Many faith traditions include a prayer or edict about being thankful for suffering; it is easy for mental health professionals to see why this is so. This suffering is a gift, a way that our bodies and psyches tell us that change is needed. All we need to do is listen to this inner voice, be patient and accepting in our comprehension, and respond.

Try as we might, there is really no way to avoid responsibility, which will always settle, like water, into a low place if that is all we aspire to. This is sometimes a hard-won lesson for many college students and their families. In the boiling kettle that is emerging adulthood, many students encounter experiences with responsibility, whether they themselves assume that responsibility or not. Some have difficulties with roommates but retreat into silence or sticky-note communications, or perhaps ask to be reassigned to another room. Some skip class too often and also try to skip out on the inevitable conversation about grades. Some overindulge in partying or any of the innumerable forms of gluttony, then pass along troubles to others through distractions and problems with sleep or health or relationships or the law. But no matter the manifestation, someone, somewhere, will always pay. Sometimes the student will pay, but maybe much, much later in life. Sometimes it is the parents who pay. Sometimes, when the water is allowed to gather in the lowest place possible, it will be someone who wasn't really expecting this but finally says "Enough!" That might be a friend, or a judicial affairs officer, or a counselor, or the court.

That teenagers and young adults attempt such maneuvering is nothing new, of course. Somewhere deep in a Spanish cave there is probably a drawing of a hungry and worried Neanderthal parent trying to rouse a hairy teen from slumber on a warm rock, as a herd of juicy beasts passes by their dwelling. Hey, at least they didn't have cell phones! This form of dodging is well known by all of us, because we all tried it and either learned the easy way or the hard way that it doesn't work too well. What does appear to be a more recent phenomenon is older adults, those who are responsible for guiding the young into successful adulthood, engaging in their own dodging, and with atrocious consequences for themselves and their charges.

Most folks who work in higher education environs can cite examples of parents who did not or could not say "Enough!" and hold their adult children responsible. Perhaps oddly, given the term, the *helicopter parent*, who hovers over schools and other systems and strikes with ferocity when the institution "didn't do its job correctly," is frequently an example of a parent who is failing to hold students responsible, especially for rather ordinary problem solving. Just as the hairy Neanderthal teen can throw a spear, so can college students pick up a telephone and assert themselves with others. Rather than use the helicopter metaphor, perhaps we should try the term *nursemaid*.

To be fair, it is not just parents who err in this way. When any of us involved in higher education (or any of our society's institutions) fail to draw a line in behavior, and fail to apply the natural consequences we ourselves would face were we to behave in a similar fashion, we engage in hurtful dodging. We enable continued unethical conduct when we let the water pass downward to someone else, perhaps even some unfortunate soul in the distant future. It takes courage for anyone, in any sector of our culture, to confront hazing, or alcohol abuse, or sexual assault, or election tampering, or hatred and bigotry. There are always those who perpetuate these social ills, and they fight us.

But confront we must. Some in higher education enable because they have difficulty watching a young person suffer in a mess of his or her own creation. Sometimes this is done in the name of "student development." This tendency is not only myopic but also dangerous, because by dodging in this way we ensure that someone, somewhere, will pay, and often with a much less attractive outcome. Students must learn directly from their own experiences, and sometimes this involves discomfort, pain, and loss. Let's not get in the way of this most precious form of learning.

A Model of College Parenting

The model of which I speak here applies to anyone who is involved in parenting, re-parenting, fostering, or supporting the college student.

Being a good parent is the toughest job in the world. Parenting involves a seemingly limitless set of skills and tasks, and it is rare that any of us was explicitly taught anything about how to perform them. We simply watch others, primarily our own parents, and model ourselves after them. But this often means we acquire both good and bad habits. All parents, even the "best" parents, make mistakes along the way. This seems to be an unavoidable part of the human condition. Nonetheless, it is possible for us to catch ourselves making these mistakes, to interrupt them, and to improve our parenting skills.

In some ways, being a good parent of a college student is even tougher. Not only are we expected (by our children, friends, society) to make good judgments across many dimensions of our young adult children's lives, we are supposed to do it from a distance, as our children are often not living in our homes while in college. They are away, yet their needs continue and are changing as they mature. Our students still need some support, and yet they are growing and should be able to provide some things for themselves. They still need us to monitor their progress somewhat, and yet they can and should supervise themselves in important ways. How much do we give? When do we withhold? How closely do we watch them? When do we let go? These are all difficult questions, to which many parents are seeking answers.

In this section I try to summarize what I have learned during 27 years as a practicing psychologist who works exclusively with college students and their families. This is not an attempt to address all parenting skill sets, because that would be an enormous, if not impossible, task. Rather, I focus on two intersecting dimensions of college parenting behavior that provide, I believe, one helpful model of decision-making and actions. Understanding this model may help us parents not only evaluate our current patterns of judgments about our students but also alter these patterns when necessary. The model also speaks to ways that higher education administrators carry out their roles in support of the developing student, and therefore is relevant to the development of IHE programs and services.

Figure 2 shows a matrix based on two axes: gratification (vertical) and supervision (horizontal). In this model gratification

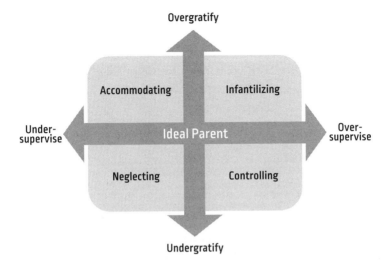

Figure 2. College Parenting Model

refers to decisions or actions to provide, withhold, or withdraw meaningful support for our student. More simply put, this refers to how much or how little we give (time, money, material possessions, etc.) as parents. Note that the top of the vertical axis refers to parents who give a lot—too much, in fact. On that end of the gratification dimension we are giving to our students when they don't need it and are capable of providing for themselves. At the bottom of this axis, we have parents who give too little. In other words, we as parents are at the bottom when our students are not capable of providing for themselves and we are not attending to this need.

For the purpose of this model, the supervision dimension, on the horizontal axis, refers to the degree to which we as parents are monitoring or watching our students' progress. Parents on the left side of the matrix are supervising too little. This occurs when we are not paying attention to our students' lives when they need our attention. At the right side of the dimension are parents who provide too much supervision. In other words, we as parents are on that side of the spectrum when are watching or controlling very closely at a time when our students do not need it; they are capable of functioning just fine without our oversight.

At the center of the matrix we have the "ideal parent." That is, we are the ideal college parent when we provide just the right amount of both gratification and supervision, neither too much nor too little, and we do it at the right time and in the right circumstances. Sounds easy, right? Well, as you already know, it isn't. Not by a long shot. It is very difficult to be ideal in these judgments. It requires that we know what our students are capable, and not capable, of doing at a particular moment in time and in a particular set of circumstances. Further, their capabilities change from time to time and situation to situation. Just how in the heck do we become ideal college parents anyway? Obviously, perfection is not possible, and we as parents shouldn't expend all our energy trying to attain it. But we can improve what we do if we just know a little about what to look for, both in our students and in ourselves.

Before we go any further, let's take a look at some assumptions that are made in this model of college parenting.

- All parents make mistakes. Sometimes we give or watch too much or too little. Accepting this fact makes it possible for us to relax and try to do better.

- Parents move around the matrix. Very few of us always give or watch too much or too little. One day we might give too much, the next too little, and so on. After all, we have bad days, too.

- The "ideal" spot on the matrix depends on the development of your student and the situation in which he finds himself. Depending on his circumstances, you may need to increase or decrease your level of gratification and supervision. The key is knowing your student and what he should be capable of doing independently.

- We can "move" toward an ideal spot on the matrix. Once you grasp the nature of your student's capabilities and her circumstances, you can engage in a decision or action that is close to an ideal spot on the matrix.

Parenting Styles

Now that we have some of the basics out of the way, let's focus on the styles of parenting that are revealed by the matrix. The two intersecting dimensions of gratification and supervision result in four parenting quadrants. These are:

- Overgratifying and oversupervising, or *infantilizing*. Parents who give and supervise too much are treating their students like infants, as though they are not capable of providing for or monitoring themselves.
- Overgratifying and undersupervising, or *accommodating*. Parents who give too much but supervise too little are simply accommodating their student, granting all her wishes without any expectations for or monitoring of her behavior.
- Undergratifying and oversupervising, or *controlling*. Parents who give very little but monitor the behavior of their student very closely don't adequately provide for his needs and appear to be more interested in controlling or managing his affairs.
- Undergratifying and undersupervising, or *neglecting*. Parents who neither provide for needs nor monitor behavior are neglecting of their student's development.

In this model, the terms *infantilizing, accommodating, controlling*, and *neglecting* are viewed as negative parenting styles because it is assumed that the style doesn't match the needs or development of the student. Parents who engage in the most extreme versions of these styles would be plotted at the corners of the matrix, and those who are less extreme would be plotted near the center. The quadrants are based upon an unspecified, hypothetical student and situation, so it is purely artificial. Only in theory should we, as parents, be "in the center" of this matrix. If our young adult is perfectly able to provide for and monitor herself, then of course we should be in the center. Obviously, many students are not yet able to do this. Therefore the ideal spot on the matrix depends on the individual student, on his capabilities, on her situation. There are times when it is appropriate for us to increase or decrease our gratification and supervision of our young adult children. When we do well in matching our responses to our students in this way, we are in effect advancing their own healthy psychological development.

Let's attempt to apply the model to real-life people and situations. (Names and other identifying information have been changed.) Read the following scenarios and try to plot the parenting style on the matrix. You might also ask yourself how you would respond to the situation, and then plot your own style on the matrix, as well.

- Chris, a 20-year-old male student, has received a D in a college class. It is his only grade below a B at this point. He is alcohol and drug free, manages his own finances well, and has never been arrested or in violation of the school's code of conduct. His parents are disappointed in the grade, but have never voiced their expectations for his performance and continue to give him more than $3,000 per month in "spending money." Due to their concern over the D, however, his mother drives four hours to campus every week to make sure he attends his therapy session. She calls to wake him every morning and calls throughout the day to make sure he has attended class and other commitments. She insists on reading his mail and paying his bills for him.

- A 19-year-old female student, Valerie, has accrued over $40,000 in debt on 17 credit cards. She is drinking alcohol excessively, and much of the money has been spent on food and alcohol for her friends, for concerts, and for traveling away from campus. Her father, a health-care professional, writes a single check to pay for the debt. There is no other action taken.

- Nikita, a 21-year-old female student, is entirely self-sufficient financially. She works 20 hours per week and pays her own tuition and rent through her income and student loans. She lives in a rickety apartment in a less-than-desirable part of town. She is often fatigued and stressed and is embroiled in conflict with a boyfriend who is using drugs and is sometimes emotionally abusive. Her father suspects the boyfriend is spending the nights with his daughter in her apartment. He installs a digital camera in her bedroom without her knowledge and consent.

- An 18-year-old male student named Ronald is living out of his vehicle and does not have enough funds to buy books or other class materials. He pulls this off for a while, but eventually the stress takes a toll and he has an emotional breakdown. He seeks help at the university, and a representative contacts the parents for support. They refuse to come to town, as they live in another state. They do call their son, and tell him to "shape up quick."

These are examples of, in order, the infantilizing, accommodating, controlling, and neglecting styles of parenting. In each case, the response provided did not match the student's capabilities or situation. Using the matrix as our guide, we can attempt to plot a more appropriate response in these examples.

- Chris needs less gratification and supervision. His D grade is not catastrophic and it is apparent he is capable of functioning well and monitoring himself. Expectations about grades should, however, be communicated.

- Valerie needs less gratification and more supervision. It is clear that her resources are more than adequate but also that she is not fully capable of managing choices on her own.

- Nikita needs more gratification and less supervision. She is independent and capable of functioning on her own but needs more resources to do it well. The supervision her father provides seems oriented more toward catching her doing something he disapproves of than being helpful to her.

- Ronald needs more gratification and supervision. His needs are being neglected entirely.

These examples represent extremes. It may be much more challenging to apply the matrix to your own young adult child. And yet it can be done. Those interested may want to start by asking themselves a few simple questions:

- What is my student capable of doing on his own?

- Is there evidence in her history of relying on her own resources? Of her monitoring her own choices and conduct?

- How does he compare with his peers in these areas? Does he seem capable of more or less than his peers? If less capable, this doesn't mean that you need to maintain high levels of support and monitoring. You may need to start high but have a plan to gradually diminish these levels as your student reaches milestones.

- How has your student handled problems or crises in the past? Did she do it well or poorly? A reasonably healthy 17- to 24-year-old should be able to manage a wide range of issues on her own.

- What has your student needed from you in the past? Did it help? Did he learn from what you gave him? What is the nature of his current situation? Is it a situation that is common or typical for young adults? Or is it something that most college students do not experience?

Now let's look at some rather ordinary situations that frequently arise with college students. Try again to think of your response to each of the following situations and plot them on the matrix. This time, assume that what follows is the only information you have about the situation. By the way, these too represent real-life situations; they have actually occurred and with some regularity.

- Your student was late on an assignment and needs to talk to the professor. She asks you to contact the professor.
- Your student is in conflict with his roommate and wants to move out of the dorm or get a new roommate.
- Your student overdrew her checking account and has a fee to pay. She asks you to put more money in the account.
- Your student was cited for underage drinking. He has a court appearance and fees to pay. He asks you to help with these responsibilities.
- Your student reveals that she only passed one of four classes this semester. It is time to register for the next semester's classes.
- Your student calls you at 11:30 p.m. to say that he has no clean clothes.
- Your student tells you that she does not know how or where to buy books.
- Your student sends you an email in which he informs you that he has a bad cold and has missed classes for two days.

All other things being equal, in each case there are actions these students need to take to meet their responsibilities or take care of their needs, and they should be able to do this with minimal supervision. Any role you take would be minor, mostly restricted to providing information (or helping them find it). It would be rarely necessary, if not ineffective, for a parent to resolve these matters instead of letting the young adult child do so.

In short, you can make an educated guess about the approach to parenting that is appropriate given your student's history and situation. If his history is such that he is capable of securing his own resources and of supervising himself independently, then you may want to decrease gratification and support. If her situation is unusual for most college students, then you may want to increase gratification and supervision. The model is flexible, so we as parents can be too. If you find that you are "off the mark," don't worry. Just regroup and make another attempt toward a different point in the matrix. Do this as often as you need. Remember, we don't have to be perfect; we just need to try and do our best. After some tweaking, that will be good enough.

Julie was raised by a single mother in a rural area. The oldest of four children, she had two brothers and a sister, the youngest. Due to their circumstances, Julie was raised to be independent and self-sufficient. She was a wee girl when she learned the basics of cooking, cleaning, and babysitting. Her mother worked the second shift in a chicken processing plant and usually did not get home until well after 8 p.m. Julie was expected to have the kids fed and bathed by then—which she did, and did well. She loved her family and was kind and giving to all of them. She did not complain when one of the others had temper tantrums or got scraped up playing outside. In the midst of all this responsibility and noise, Julie somehow got all of her homework done. To others she seemed quiet, perhaps sullen at times, but they also noticed a steely resolve and competence in nearly everything she tried. She once stared down a bully in the schoolyard, never making a threat or striking out in any way. Julie simply stood her ground and locked gazes with him. She did not budge, and eventually the boy slinked away with his confederates.

Julie was smart and everyone knew it. She made top grades and read all the books that were in her meager middle school library. Along the way she even helped a couple of friends with their homework and tests. Her aura was that of a star, and she led everyone to think that this was just who she was, that it was all natural and with no real larger purpose. But actually, and very privately, Julie wanted to leave. She wanted to see other parts of the world and taste other experiences, and she knew, since her mother often reminded her, that there would be no money for college and that her brains provided her with the only means of making her dream a reality. This dream was like a hot coal burning in her breast, and she tended to it every day. It is with such resolutions that stubbornness becomes a virtue, among the finest traits human beings can possess.

The arc of Julie's life continued without interruption. In high school her success picked up pace, partly due to the family imperative of independence taking root in her now older siblings, but mostly due to her unfettered intelligence. Julie would become the valedictorian, she thought. And she did. She also was a leader in several school and church activities, representing her area in girls' state and regional math and science competitions. She won two of these in her final year. By then her mother had begun making wisecracks about boys and dating. Julie stared these down too, but her mother did not slink off as easily as the bully. "I don't have time for that, Mom," she would say, sharply. Julie did not countenance any form of criticism. She'd been a good daughter—no, a great daughter, and she knew it. She'd been a good kid, too; she excelled at things and caused no heartburn for anyone in her life. Julie knew this combination was rare and that she would be a very hot property to many. "I will be able to go to any school I want," she often said to herself.

This turned out to be true. She received many offers and scholarships, not a small number including a full ride: tuition, books, supplies, housing—the works. Julie chose a well-known and respected private school in another state and continued her customarily stellar performance there. The school had a formal past affiliation with a religious denomination, one with which she familiar through her family and church. It suited her for these reasons. Julie sailed through her first year as content as she ever had been; more so, really, because she did not have any of her former obligations. During her sophomore year, she explored more of what the school had to offer in the social arena, which she enjoyed very much. Julie learned she could enjoy friendships, and more importantly, these did not seem to impede her progress in the least. There were, of course, the usual distractions and temptations, but she much preferred being firmly in control, so for her there was no appeal in such things. In the winter of that year she learned something that took her by surprise, unsettling her fine-tuned sense of order and control.

Julie liked girls. She liked boys too, but not exactly in the same way. Except perhaps for the circumstances of her birth, she'd been blessed with good fortune her whole life, and this continued once she had barely opened her eyes, peeked around a bit, and found love—or you might say, love found her, as her partner was the one who did the pursuing. Julie had always been the caregiver, but now it had become her time to enjoy some of the best things the world has to offer. Not for one second did she waste the opportunity. This was the happiest time of her life.

Then her mother found out. Someone at school, unknown to Julie, had contacted her mother and told her about the romance. Not once in Julie's life had her mother withdrawn her support or attempted to control her in any way beyond appropriate safety concerns for children. Thus it shocked Julie when her mother showed up, unannounced on campus, and told her that she was withdrawing her from school and bringing her home. "Get in the car," she bleated. "Or what?" Julie replied. In tears, her mother cried, "Or you'll never see your brothers and sister again!" Shaking, Julie ran off to hide. She texted her partner about what had happened, and a little later they met to console each other as best they could.

Julie already vaguely knew she couldn't be withdrawn against her will, and this was confirmed by the counselor whom she had called that afternoon. She also knew that her funding source was secure and had nothing to do with her mother. Unbeknownst to Julie, her mother had gone to the campus police department and was frustrated to learn that officers were not able or willing to detain Julie, who had not broken the law or violated any campus policy. Still, Julie was mortified at the prospect of not seeing her siblings. Many days passed before she spoke to her mother again, and during this time Julie missed classes for the first time. This created a panic the likes of which she had never known. She did not know what to do.

After talking with a counselor, someone in the dean of students' office, a campus minister, and her resident assistant, Julie learned that the panic belonged to her mother. It took some weeks, but she also realized that no one could stop her from having a relationship with her siblings, though her mother might try to interfere. With time she regained her equilibrium and was better able to focus on class again. Julie had endured a situation in which her economic support was stable, but emotional support was withdrawn or threatened. This pattern affected the balance of gratification she needed to function well as a student. She had also rather suddenly moved from a status of minimal supervision over her life to a foreboding sense that someone was watching and reporting on her activities. Both axes of college parenting had teetered and left her knocked off center in terms of her baseline functioning. This disruption had affected her studies, though thanks to her many psychological resources, the disruption was brief. Even so, the episode left her with additional psychic burdens she had not had before: a need to reconcile matters with her mother and preserve all the family connections that were dear to her. Julie was certain she would do well in class, but she also knew these burdens would take months or longer to resolve. Not all of her energy, therefore, could be devoted to her primary tasks, growing and learning.

Determining Local Expectations and Preparedness for Meeting Them

It isn't just parents who facilitate or hobble growth and learning; all campus personnel may in one way or another serve as parental surrogates. Colleges must act with keen awareness of factors that promote or impair learning and that offer the best possible balances of gratification and supervision of a wide variety of students. In addition to gathering information about campus and community mental health needs and resources, as defined in Chapter 2, administrators would do well to investigate the landscape of societal pressures in their area. This requires stepping outside familiar territory, such as the fiscal one, to consider the universe of expectations bearing on their campuses. The views of all stakeholders must be reviewed—students, faculty, staff, parents, donors—with attention to diversity and inclusion. Nearly all schools conduct some form of needs assessment, satisfaction, or outcome research, and these are good data, but very few extrapolate how *realistic* the results may be or what any departure from reality may mean about the community. This departure will tell you a lot about unhealthy pressures brought to bear on students, and what types of distress students are likely to feel.

As you formulate questions to ask, it is helpful to categorize them into *aspirations, shoulds,* and *musts,* with the last likely representing the most acute sources of distress. The resulting profile will vary, sometimes wildly, from school to school. The questions should be phrased as follows: "What do I think that Campus U (hopefully will, should, must) provide to me?" and "What do I think that Campus U (hopefully will, should, must) provide to the campus community?" One can do this in an open-ended response style, or one can ask respondents to choose from among keywords they will then match to one of the three response categories. The keywords may be rationally derived from what is already known about local circumstances, or they may be produced in focus groups brainstorming about local pinch points. Here are some keywords that may be applicable:

- Status or image
- Avoiding stigma
- Employment
- Income
- A meaningful life
- Social connections
- Return on investment
- Social justice
- Preservation of privilege
- Good grades
- Fidelity to family and their beliefs
- Contentment with career
- Clear pathways to advancement
- Entertainment
- Amenities and comforts
- Minimal disruption
- Challenge
- Support for development
- Teaching independence
- Teaching community
- Marketable skills
- Life skills
- Safety
- Adventure

And so on. It would be all fine and good, laudable even, if these were merely aspirations of community members. But no school can provide all of these as imperatives; they must choose where to place their energy and resources. Universities will do well on some, a yeoman's job on some, and poorly on some. Any veteran politician will tell you that you can't please everyone. What follows, then, is a rational assessment of how well the school performs on items like these. A logical source of information about that may be the school's complaint process, perhaps through an online format. This should provide a picture or heat map of the areas in which there is the most intensity, provided that the complaint process is oriented toward or accounts for the goals outlined here.

Let's say you've done this and now are wondering what the mental health "heat map" may look like. Walking through the list again, we see some hypotheses about that. Remember, the issues will in theory result from an *overemphasis* on the imperative.

- Status or image (anxiety, perfectionism)
- Avoiding stigma (fear, isolation)
- Employment (anxiety, competitiveness)
- Income (drive, meaninglessness)
- A meaningful life (confusion, misdirection, angst)
- Social connections (social anxiety, time and stress management)
- Return on investment (robotism, depression)
- Social justice (anger, guilt, fear)
- Preservation of privilege (obliviousness, protectionism)
- Good grades (anxiety, lack of true learning, academic stagnation)
- Fidelity to family and their beliefs (insulation, loss of identity and gifts)
- Contentment with career (unidimensional living)
- Clear pathways to advancement (blind ambition)
- Entertainment (poor distress tolerance, poor work ethic)
- Amenities and comforts (depression, lack of risk taking)
- Minimal disruption (lack of growth, depression)
- Challenge (anxiety, avoidance, stagnation)
- Support for development (lack of creativity and independence)

- Teaching independence (isolation, poor relationships)
- Teaching community (anxiety, obsession with approval)
- Marketable skills (robotism, meaninglessness, depression)
- Life skills (dependence, lack of spontaneity)
- Safety (fear, anxiety, isolation)
- Adventure (lack of rhythm and routine, stress)

Once an IHE determines its profile, it can assess how prepared it is to manage these pressures. This will involve a review not only of resources but also of the prevailing paradigms from which it operates and how well those match the heat maps. Many times they do not, and this sets the stage for brokenness in the community's response to needs. The college will also need a thorough review of branding, image, and marketing activities to determine how these may be facilitating or mitigating campus pressures and their mental health sequelae. As but one example, it has been noted that a school's competitive climate had an unintended though direct bearing on rates of distress, depression, and suicide (Blidner, 2015). Adjustments to those elements, along with a concerted effort to change campus culture, were undertaken to reduce those outcomes. The fact is, every school ought regularly to investigate its own gifts, as well as its brokenness, striving to enhance the former and minimize the latter.

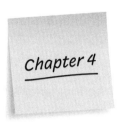

Chapter 4

Orientation Mismatch and Young Adults' Needs

The psychological development of the late adolescent and young adult is complex and riddled with emotional volatility, critical incidents, relationship turmoil, and the fits and starts of the search for identity and autonomy. Every IHE that seeks to produce competent learners and citizens should ideally facilitate the growth of the self in its students. It is only through contact with and expression of a student's genuine self that it, and the students it serves, can claim any lasting success. But the psychic landscape of the young is pocked with landmines, which any college can inadvertently trigger, if it is not paying attention to these factors and to its local campus culture.

When service paradigms and models are chosen by default—or worse, randomly and chaotically—such triggering is inevitable. The school can find itself unwittingly creating and perpetuating the very situations over which it may groan the loudest. As noted in the previous chapter, the imperatives of its constituents will lead to negative outcomes if one is unconscious or thoughtless about them. We now turn our attention to these dynamics as they relate to students' mental health needs and the services intended to address them.

Loss of Privacy and Autonomy

It may not be well known to those outside higher education that there is a tremendous amount of energy behind the search for information concerning college students. From vendors to credit card companies to judicial networks to administrators and parents, myriad individuals and entities want the skinny on students. Sometimes the desire is based in altruistic and other well-intentioned motives; sometimes it is decidedly not. Even when the motives are healthy, very few understand the impact of this search on the campus mental health service and, more importantly, on the student seeking mental health services.

Students, like all consumers, want value for their time and dollar. They are, in my experience, pretty savvy customers and fairly merciless when they are disappointed with the service they receive. Outfits that deign to provide those services had better well have some magic in their goods, or the student will be out the door before they know what hit them. And therein lies the problem for college counseling centers.

One could argue that there is an enormous amount of value in mental health services, and one would be correct. The opportunity to learn about the self, to manifest authentic and healthy adulthood, to remedy past trauma, to have a healing relationship, and to live free of terrible symptoms are wondrous gifts provided by skilled hands. But the average college student does not, probably cannot, see this at the outset and sometimes even after a while. It's difficult for anyone to fathom life in the absence of pain, or the beauty of what it is like to be a genuine self. Oh, but what they can see is the gift of privacy, of having at least one place in their lives where they can say what they want and try out various selves until they find one that fits. College students can see this even before they dial the center's number or visit the office itself. It will be clear to them in advertisements and in the physical orientation of the office; it will be clear to them within minutes of entering the facility and of talking with a therapist; and it will be increasingly obvious as the service negotiates through requests and demands for information about them. This privacy, this sanctuary, is the essential magic of mental health services, the magic that breeds all other magic the services can provide. Without it, no other benefits accrue; it is the oxygen of therapy and change. Even the slightest ill-considered breach of this boundary can be fatal to healing, though students generally understand when good communication is necessary.

All others in the student's life simply must understand this. Everyone, from a police officer to a dean, must respect this fundamental truth if they have an interest in the developmental goals of students. In the overwhelming majority of situations, the goals of society and institutions are not that different from the goals of students; there is a great deal of overlap. If you tamper with or take away this magic, a vacuum is created, and positive growth is stunted or terminated. A simple but oft-overlooked principle is to ask the student for the information you want. Allow him or her the autonomy and self-determination that is embedded in our federal constitution: life, liberty, and the pursuit of happiness.

Special Considerations concerning Mental Health Records

As medicine has adopted electronic records systems and pushed for integrated health care operations (the actual working definition of which varies widely), concerns about privacy and oversharing records have arisen (Davenport, 2017). A recent Google search for this erosion of privacy resulted in 97,600,000 hits. In 2015, an estimated 100 million health care records were stolen, affecting approximately one in three Americans, an increase of 11,000% over the previous year. In South Carolina, 13 hospital employees were fired over privacy breaches (*Insurance Journal*, 2018). Clearly, security has not kept pace with developments in the technology involved (Costello, 2016). This situation is ripe for lawsuits.

Some have warned that such records systems can lead to other types of damages, pointing to 147 such adverse events in 2013 alone, and have clearly advised for the separation of physical and mental health records (Thomas, 2014). There has also been a successful movement in Minnesota that is using legislation to challenge forced shared records adoption by psychologists in health-care settings (Huey, 2016). Its leaders cite two main motivations: potential for harm and the right of psychologists to govern their own practices.

As if this was not of enough concern, some of these operational models, which may include mental health services, also build in compulsory "consent" to share records with unnamed "health-care professionals." I say compulsory because this consent is required in order to receive services. This consent process occurs when one is under the duress of suffering and before one can know what exactly is in the record, the purpose of the sharing, and who will receive it. This means that such a process fails to secure informed consent, part of the ethical bedrock of the mental health professions, something we learn almost from the moment we set foot in training programs.

In all 50 states, clients of a variety of mental health professionals are granted the right of privileged communication in therapy. Aside from exceptions having to do with harm to self or others, this right is absolute; no third party is entitled to receive this information. Compulsory consent processes force therapy clients to waive the right of privilege in toto; once it is waived, there is no longer any privilege. No other professional services for which persons may claim privilege (clergy, attorneys) engage in compulsory consent in order to receive their assistance—because it is ethically and morally wrong to do so.

In addition to the violation of informed consent and right of privilege, these practices fail to respect the autonomy of persons, their right to self-determination and choice. They also fail to act with integrity, beneficence, and nonmaleficence in carrying out professional services. These duties are spelled out in the ethical codes of all mental health professions in one way or another. There is a repeated avoidance of addressing these vital ethical, legal, and consumer concerns in discussions of integrated care programs (Polychronis, 2018). For example, it is alarming to see how the psychology profession in particular is so eager to abandon these core foundations of the psychologist-client relationship in order, basically, to get in on the ground floor of the integrated-care trend. Frequently, these ethical matters are either sidestepped entirely, or there are poorly founded campaigns to change existing ethical codes and laws, which are now framed as outmoded obstacles to integrated care that must be circumvented (Polychronis, 2018).

Compulsory and total consent processes are presumably sought after for two reasons: perceived ease of communication and the convenience of business procedures, including billing (in all honesty, I think the latter is the real motivation). It is claimed that such conveniences result in improved outcomes, but research support for such a conclusion is mixed. Where support exists, it regards those who cannot speak for themselves, such as the very young, the very old, and those who have been deemed incompetent. It is an injustice to treat all persons in this same manner. Further, an informed consent process at the point information is needed has always been available. In 27 years of practice, I have never known this to not work well.

Combine lack of security with totally open mental health records and you have an enormous problem. Oversharing and failure to respect persons will lead to injury and therefore litigation, which is one way to resolve these predicaments. The media will also get involved, and that is another potential pathway to resolution. Or we could all just go ahead and do the right thing.

After several challenging attempts at learning how to be in a relationship, Robert was delighted to have a new girlfriend. In the past he had been too clumsy, or too demanding, and some of his exes had been too avoidant or too rushed. By now he had grown in his own self-understanding, and this made him a better friend to others, including and perhaps especially to women whom he was interested in dating. Robert had experiences in which he felt guilt for being unclear at times, too pushy at times, and too lazy or passive at others. Early on, he did not know who he was as a partner or what exactly he expected from romance or sex. With his first partners, he felt he had made every mistake in the book, and either the women involved or life itself showed him what did and what did not work well. But he was observant and introspective to a degree, so he paid attention and learned his lessons.

Robert was raised in the context of evangelical Christianity, which, as far as relationships go, mainly taught him through an aura of taboo and control of sinful impulses. He enjoyed many things about his upbringing, but he privately dismissed much of this teaching, seeing how the adults often did not seem to follow their own strictures. His family was not that different from others in his area; they had their share of affairs and other peccadilloes, divorces, and the occasional unwanted birth. Somewhere along the way he figured he could do better just by setting off on his own—which he did, and did well, carefully managing his own privacy within his family and community. Robert was finding his way in the world in ways that usually worked for himself and for others, too. He felt good that he had tried to do the right thing and never purposefully hurt anyone, while having a good amount of fun along the way.

Of all the women he had dated, he learned the most from Tina. She was a force of nature, one to be reckoned with for sure, but he liked her feistiness, her energy, her white-hot passions. She did everything at breakneck speed, and watching her was like watching a bottle rocket with a short fuse. Tina left a trail of suspense-filled awe behind her. In keeping with her style she was sexually aggressive, and Robert had no problem with this whatsoever. It was with her that he learned he genuinely enjoyed a more passive role, in no small part because it alleviated any feelings of responsibility for the activity or its outcome. At times he liked not having to think about such things. Of course this meant risk, but Robert was just beginning to enjoy thrills, in contrast with the very safe life he had lived before college. With Tina he felt that all the risks they took were worthwhile because neither one of them got hurt; nor did they get emotionally attached to each other or experience the anxiety that often comes with closeness. Or so he thought.

In truth, Tina did give him one lasting problem, which it took quite some time for him to figure out; he went through two subsequent girlfriends and was currently on his third before he discovered it. Robert had chlamydia. Asymptomatic for many months, he had only recently noticed symptoms, causing him to visit his campus nurse. The college was small and did not have a lab or a full-time physician on staff. They had to refer off campus for many services. In keeping with standards of medical confidentiality, and its terms of consent, the campus health service referred Robert to both a local lab and a urologist. His lab results and chart notes arrived at the urologist's office within 24 hours of his visit, before he was informed of the referral. This was all well and good, and *might* have worked well in a large city, but this occurred in a small one, one in which the aunt of Robert's girlfriend worked in the urologist's office. The health service did not know that—couldn't have known it. Not even Robert knew, though later he might have guessed.

The aunt was an administrative assistant in the physician's office. She performed a wide range of clerical duties, including scheduling, billing, managing files, and processing referrals, in both directions to and from the office. She saw Robert's information in the course of these tasks and knew he dated her niece. Strictly speaking, it could be argued that she did not violate privacy law because she did not disclose specific private health information, but she did warn her niece to stay away from Robert. The niece pressed her aunt for more information but none was forthcoming. Ultimately, because they were family and each respected the other, the end came to the relationship with Robert. And he never knew why. He just got a cold text one day, and his girlfriend stopped responding to him thereafter. He was hurt, but he'd been through this before, so it did not seem unusual in the world of twenty-somethings. Robert moved on. He was quickly treated and sent on to live his life as he wanted to. Everything seemed normal.

Except it wasn't. What had occurred was theft. It wasn't his records that were stolen, not exactly anyway. It was his autonomy, or the ability to manage his own affairs, that had been taken from him, and Robert was in no way incompetent in that area. In two separate acts of paternalism, Robert's life was needlessly altered and in ways that were not made known to him. If the law was not broken, its spirit certainly was. Less arguable is the ethics or morality of this story. All competent adults, and I think emerging adults in particular, ought to be treated with respect and given the opportunity to make choices concerning their personal information. Acting in this way also provides individuals with valuable learning opportunities in many dimensions of life, including the most intimate, such as sexuality and relationships. When individuals or systems interfere with learning, no matter how legally "justifiable" the interference may be, they do young adults a serious disservice.

How could this story have unfolded differently? First, Robert could have been given the opportunity to have fully informed consent about the release of his records. He could then have known more about the travel of his information and what persons would have access to it. Second, though a nurse did tell Robert "to be careful" with his partners, he could have been more firmly directed to inform them or take other precautions against infection. (In this tale, there is no guarantee that his partner, and perhaps others, was already infected, but no one could know that.) Robert could have been referred to counseling for this purpose;

therapists are skilled in these kinds of conversations. No matter where he was treated, Robert should have spoken to his partners, including the one who had likely infected him. Doing so may even have neutralized any problem with the treating medical office. Third, and perhaps most critical, Robert could have been counseled about risky sexual practices, or, more to the point in terms of his growth trajectory, the risks of being too passive in relationships. These steps might have transformed a disaster into a priceless lesson of life, affecting his whole future in a positive way.

Failing to Listen

So there's a great little video called *It's Not about the Nail* out in the electronic ether, all about the importance of listening (Headley, 2013). Watching it, one thinks about relationship contexts mainly, especially the oft-seen tendency of men to fix things instead of just empathizing and supporting their partners.

Ah, but the video is a great object lesson for professional helpers. There is a strong sense of urgency among many health-care providers to quickly and efficiently apply the "intervention" to the "symptom," because that is what the diagnosing/insurance/billing industrial complex demands. The forces behind this complex are tremendous and so embedded in some helping systems that many don't stop and think for a moment about how this form of "helping" may be affecting the "helped."

Sometimes it doesn't matter how "right" the helper is. The one receiving the help must feel heard and understood first, as this facilitates acceptance and motivation to be helped in the first place. I recall a story about a homeless woman, hungry and cold, who upbraided a good Samaritan for "throwing me a bone." Before she received food and clothing, she wanted to be understood, to be treated like a human being. In particular she wanted her pain to be understood. That was her primary need at the moment. Her "helpers" assumed her physical needs were more fundamental than her emotional or spiritual needs. This is where many of us go awry.

The video takes us back to the early days of our training. We were first taught basic helping skills, such as empathy, genuineness, positive regard, and active listening. Somehow the systems we work in may distract us from these elemental approaches to human suffering. Let's go back then, and learn this all over again. If you are involved in training the next generation of helpers, consider showing them the video. After the jokes subside, tell them to get serious about this one.

Listening involves much more than the ears. Our therapeutic ancestors told us to develop a "third ear," the ability to perceive behind the words and nonverbal behavior the essence of a client's story and predicament. Failing to do this can result in our unknowingly adding to or reinforcing the client's problems. One example of such iatrogenesis is the facilitation of an *illness identity*. This can occur when the practitioner recursively interprets the universe of client experience as reflective of the condition or illness being treated, and feeding this perception back to the client as a form of narrative of the client's life. Lichstein (2017) has demonstrated this phenomenon in cases of reported insomnia in which the client's perception of illness has become "uncoupled" from actual sleep. The author defines an illness identity as the "conviction" that one has an illness in the absence of supporting facts. He estimates that up to 25% of cases of insomnia are accounted for by this phenomenon! This is one heavy cost of failing to listen or being in a hurry.

At the end of her math class, Susan realized she had not heard a single thing her instructor said. She liked him as a teacher, thought him clever and funny in all the right ways, but she recalled nothing about what had happened in class. She would later dismiss this episode, mumbling to herself that maybe it was due to her fitful sleep the night before. Susan trudged on as before, and the memory soon faded. A couple of weeks later, she couldn't find her car keys. A friend rescued her from the frenzy that followed, texting that her keys were at her place, reminding Susan that they partied there recently. "I didn't drink that much," she thought, which was true—this time. That same week the math episode happened again. She began wondering what was wrong, as this was very unlike her. She knew herself, as did her friends, to be a very organized person, someone who "had it all together"—so much so that others sought out her counsel from time to time.

Susan's anxiety grew when some less-than-stellar grades began trickling in, and not just from her math class; two other classes were also affected. A dull panic set in as older fears were resurrected from her middle-school years, when she had labored under feelings of inadequacy. Susan didn't mention this to anyone, especially her mother, who had enough troubles of her own. She didn't enjoy talking to her mother these days because she often felt worse afterward. Her panic turned to reflexive action, one of her customary responses, when a friend talked of her experiences with stimulant treatment of ADHD. In short order Susan found a physician at the campus health center, who explained that she would have to be tested in order to receive such medication. This was arranged but would take a month to complete, and the semester would be nearly over by then. Seeing that she was distraught, he arranged for a consult with one of the health center's counselors. The physician wanted to know if the testing was contraindicated in any way. It was not. In the 20-minute session the counselor asked Susan about her academic and psychiatric history, both of which were not remarkable, except that she had always done well. Her personal life was also lacking in any explanatory detail. Relationships appeared intact and functional. He asked about her family, and Susan said "They're parents, you know? They're OK I guess." There was no history of mental illness or addictions on either side of her family, as far as Susan knew.

The testing showed what was in fact real, that Susan was experiencing detectable problems with attention, concentration, and forgetfulness. She was diagnosed with ADHD-Inattentive Type, as the diagnostic criteria had recently changed, and this diagnosis was easier to apply. Susan was prescribed Adderall, and later Vyvanse, due to initially heightened anxiety and insomnia. Her dosage was increased once, but she did not notice changes aside from being able to stay up later and, seemingly, study for longer periods. Her grades improved somewhat, but by this time she was taking different and easier classes. She'd started drinking more because she found alcohol helped her to fall asleep faster. Then, a heated argument with her mother brought her, in tears, to counseling.

Over the course of a month or so Susan revealed much anger toward her parents, especially her father. She felt very much caught in the middle with them, as her mother had been seeking her support for an estrangement from her husband. "I think he's cheating on me," she would say, adding whatever gory detail she may have discovered or thought she had discovered. Susan loved her father, in no small part because of his leadership in the community and in their Roman Catholic church. Susan also knew her mother had a somewhat histrionic flair and was prone to hyperbole, which she found aggravating. She was stunned to learn that her father was moving out and a divorce was imminent. So stunned and devastated that, for a time, Susan coped through avoidance and denial. This intensified when her father came out as gay. In her current state and developmental stage, Susan was simply overwhelmed, ashamed, and incapable of processing this information. Precious psychic energy was drained away from other tasks and roles in her life, causing her issues with attention and memory.

Susan "met the criteria" for ADHD yet did not have it. Her attention and memory problems were very real, nonetheless. Her problem was more about her inability to articulate her feelings while simultaneously suppressing intense shame and anger. This took time to unravel and ran counter to her own sense of urgency, borne of fear of failure. Susan herself pressed others to act quickly, and the system cooperated within its limits. All therapy must at times be guided by such questions as "What information is being withheld?" "What insight does the client have, or not have?" "When will the client trust me enough to share the deepest pain?" Susan offered clues to such things, but many hours of listening were required to uncover them fully. Her articulation had to be actively guided through patient and responsive listening. A healing system must have this capability built into its services, else it misses the mark. The capability requires not only keen ears but also the time it takes to do this form of listening. It is not an actuarial, content-driven exercise, in which symptoms are checked off and placed into neat categories in the style of manualized treatment. This is not to say that such approaches have no place in healing; they do, but mostly for "neat" problems, which match the "neat" inclusion criteria in the studies that support them. Most human problems are not neat in the least. This is why patient listening is so needed—as is time. Plenty of time.

Being in a Hurry

Ty Cobb was once asked to describe baseball. After a moment's pause he said "It's something like a war." There is something like a war occurring in professional mental health communities, most recently rekindled by the debates on the development of the *DSM-5*, a diagnostic manual. See a *Scientific American* blog series on this issue for more information (Wickelgren, 2012). This war has many fronts, from economic if not downright mercenary (involving the coding of disorders and therefore billing of encounters), to treatment (given connections to the pharmaceutical industry), to, perhaps most broadly, a starkly contrasting view of human beings and their problems (Cosgrove, 2010, and Doward, 2013, respectively). In this writer's humble view, nowhere is this contrast more palpable or consequential than in college mental health settings.

Late adolescents and early adults exist in the throes of a volatile period of human development. As I have mentioned previously, their psyches are roiling with energy, bubbling over as they experiment with identity in their search to find authenticity and manifest their real selves in the world. Anyone who remembers those years can resonate with this time, marked by fear, various forms of aggression, behavioral instability, relationship conflict, and academic or career missteps. This volatility is quite simply inherent in—indeed, necessary to—growth. As any parent knows, it takes a lot of patience for outsiders to see this process through, to support but also avoid negatively contaminating it in some way. Contaminating development can send youth off on an unintended, unnecessary, and possibly harmful life trajectory. Forces that discourage or abort patience in work with youth stoke the flames of warfare between developmentally and medically oriented disciplines.

To address any temptation toward dichotomous thinking or polarization, which seems so rife in society today, let me be clear. Medicine as a thoughtful profession and considered practice is a wonderful thing, capable of using its massive powers to alleviate human suffering and facilitate human growth. No one in their right mind can rationally argue otherwise. But any thoughtless or unconsidered practice is capable of great harm, no matter the profession. Recently, the former chair of the

DSM-IV Task Force, Allen Frances, who is himself a physician, wrote a brief essay on the harm caused by misdiagnosing and mislabeling (Frances, 2012). He wisely counsels caution and patience in this process. Unfortunately, those individuals and entities who stand to make a great deal of money from the industry are working in the opposite direction. Their apparent purpose is to transform medicine's grand promise into a ghastly and speedy intervention-delivery system, which may result in incorrectly pathologizing, hospitalizing, or medicating consumers— or worse. In a breathtaking development, one vendor advocates utilizing instruments to render diagnoses in three minutes and reducing one's mental health status to a single number (Post, Snyder, Byer, & Hurowitz, 2018)!

Given the complexities of college student life and development, I don't know how anyone, with any tool or level of experience, can accurately diagnose youth in three minutes—or in 10 to 15 minutes, the average duration of many medical encounters. It takes time to understand the bubbling psyches of young and old alike. Susie and Johnnie may meet "the criteria" others establish for disorder X, but that may not in any but the most cursory way capture the essence of what is happening with them. This hypothesis does not compute in those who want fast and efficient delivery of products. Susie may be caught in a cycle of fear and anger based in years of psychological torment in family dynamics, which she cannot even articulate in hours and hours of encounters. Johnnie may have difficulty focusing due to years of exposure to video games and substance use, the latter of which he hides from others, and the anger he feels toward his father, who abandoned him.

Susie and Johnnie deserve our time and attention, our best effort in creating environments that encourage them to tell their stories and be healed. Let's support and fund those efforts that provide such environments.

Jim had cycled through many offices since he was 12 years old. Principals, disciplinary and detention officers, physicians, therapists, ministers, even a cop or two—he'd seen them all. The source of their interest in him was his behavior, described as shy but aggressive and belligerent. Days or weeks would go by with Jim fading into the shadows, drawing no attention to himself whatsoever. Were it not for his occasional outbursts, many would have had no recall of him at all. Then, seemingly out of the blue, he would deck a student in the hallway or randomly damage the light fixtures at the rear of the gymnasium. By age 15 he was smoking and drinking, sometimes at school and sometimes not at school when he should have been in class. When Jim sat down with various authorities he was practically noncommunicative. He'd stare off into space and would respond, if at all, in monosyllables. The adults were interested in stopping his behavior, and he knew it. They would throw whatever was in their armamentarium at him— parent conferences, more detention, community service, medications, behavior therapy, you name it. It made no difference. They all knew the what, but none knew the why, including Jim himself.

The thing was, Jim was smart—at least, analytically smart, and in particular in math and sciences. He could skip school and still turn in more than passing homework, and he did the same in his exams. Just before his high school graduation, college and scholarship offers started to roll in from out-of-state schools especially—which is exactly what he wanted. He once told a classmate that he hated his home, his hometown, and the state he lived in, although he'd hardly seen any of the state. He wanted out and had no plans to return. And so leave he did; he accepted a nice offer from a STEM program several states away and would start there in the fall.

Almost immediately, Jim noticed a stark contrast between himself and other college students. He did not have and couldn't seem to make any friends. Jim also could not regulate his schedule in any coherent way, often staying in bed and watching videos. His academic habits continued, however, and he had no problem passing his classes or better. This too seemed different from what he heard other students describe; if they missed classes, they didn't do well. The extent of his social life revolved around getting hammered with casual acquaintances, most of whom were rich enough to supply him with alcohol and, by now, harder substances too. It was during such unbridled consumption that he met a young woman who caught his eye, and vice versa. They later swapped texts and studied together a few times. Then Jim unloaded both barrels on her by vomiting his whole life's story, thinking that she seemed to really care for him. This was a psychological overdose, which frightened her to the point of withdrawal. As was characteristic of Jim, anger followed, this time in the form of an extended blackout during which he spoke of suicide to his drinking buddies. He forthwith spent a couple of days in the local hospital. And, in a repeat of what had happened in the past, he was called before the dean of students and referred for counseling. For some time the outcome of this was also the same—that is, no outcome at all.

Jim did not realize that he had finally met his match. His therapist was seasoned, a tough woman who had no truck with any nonsense. Still, she realized that he would brook no full-frontal assault and that she would have to be patient with him; there would be no shortcuts in prying loose his secrets. Many months passed as she worked to collect information about Jim's patterns, a hard thing indeed when the party involved will not speak. She found him to have an autistic quality, often zoning out in sessions and sometimes shutting down completely. His defensive rigidity required a medical intervention, but this time she wanted him to know why he needed medication. One day she told him his thoughts and perceptions were "off," that he needed help in seeing things accurately, especially in his relationships. The pain he felt over social frustrations and the loss of a girlfriend primed him to hear this message. Shortly thereafter, Jim started new medications, and for the first time in his life was compliant in the treatment, though there was some minor slippage at the start. He began to loosen.

You'd have to call what followed a mixture of fits and starts, two steps forward and two steps backward. The ratio improved over time, and Jim's therapist could eventually detect a generally upward trajectory. Jim became more focused and talkative in sessions. She even saw him smile and crack jokes at times. He also described, almost unconsciously, engaging in healthy social behavior that did not involve loss of consciousness. "That does make me feel better," he would say. But for some, well-being is an elusive wraith, and Jim regressed several times during his therapy. He returned to substance abuse many times when he wanted to escape the responsibility of attachment, of being a good friend. His pattern was to scare the daylights out of people he said he cared about. The therapist reflected, "If this ain't anger I don't know what is."

An event subsequently took place that solidified the therapist's point of view. Back at home, Jim again severely frightened others, this time his family, through a disastrous binge that occasioned another hospital visit. Yet this time he was communicating loudly and specifically to his family, albeit in a passive-aggressive manner. In a desperate phone call to his therapist, Jim's mother said, "I think he hates us." As odd as it may seem to the layperson, and likely to many who had tried to work with Jim in the past, this was fantastic news! Jim's therapist now had a bit of a purchase on what was causing Jim's pain and could finally begin to work on it more directly. So gentle confrontations began through the formation of a tentative narrative that more closely matched Jim's life story, one that at least partially explained the need for his behavior, as self-defeating as it was. "You are angry, and you have the right to be," she wagered. Correctly. From here they knitted together a tale of deep-seated multigenerational trauma of the worst variety. Jim had gotten the least bit of a foothold on the why of his behavior, one that did not involve well-worn condemnation and punishment.

Students often need time to form and articulate a story. Often, those individuals and systems that proffer help offer a great many things, except for time. Though efficient service delivery may have its place, the process of forming a narrative is mostly not an efficient enterprise. Providing this service may be expensive in terms of time, but it need not be otherwise costly, if the paradigm and model allows for it. Most college counseling centers are able to offer services for free or with very limited fees compared to what is offered in the general marketplace. In fact, college is one of the last settings in which this golden opportunity may be provided. Given the potential costs related to student behavior, IHEs should do all they can to preserve it.

Meaninglessness and a Vacuum in Ethics

Recently *USA Today College* ran a nice little piece concerning ethics in college (Schulman, 2012). The author, Miriam Schulman, assistant director of the Markkula Center for Applied Ethics at Santa Clara University, posed five simple questions for students to consider:

- What is college worth to me?
- How can I live with someone I don't like?
- How far will I go to be accepted?

- Should I tell on someone who is doing something I think is wrong?
- Is casual sex going to be part of my life?

Wonderful questions. College life offers so many rich academic and personal experiences—so many, in fact, that it is easy to lose sight of fundamental questions we all must face in our lives: Why am I here, and what am I going to do with my life? From where I sit, working closely with students, many issues and problems could be averted and many lives enhanced through an active search for answers to these questions. I believe Socrates said so way back in the misty past.

Students and their families today focus on the practicalities of college life. They rightfully ponder where their students will live, what they will study, how will they spend their time, how will they make friends, and of course how they are going to pay for it all. These are questions that need responses, but the inquiry should not stop there, and all too often it does. Without the bigger responses to bigger questions, students often live incongruently with their genuine identities and values. They associate with people they don't truly respect and engage in activities that are meaningless or even harmful to them, which may result in a résumé packed with awesomeness but revealing experiences of little or poor quality. A competent employer will see this instantly.

Parents and administrators should spend time, ideally well before the student arrives, mulling over the big questions. Set a target, well ahead in time and space, about where students might like to land and explore their existence. One doesn't travel to another part of the world without having some sense of how one will live after arrival. Why in the world would we cheat our future selves by not doing the same thing before our college and career journeys begin?

When asked what her plans were for college, Mary Anne would always say the same thing: "I plan to make friends and have fun." She shrugged when her father reminded her that college provides an education, for which he and her mother would pay. And off she would go, merrily skipping along to her next adventures, without any apparent reaction by her father—or anyone else for that matter. Mary Anne had always been a good kid, and she knew it. She made good grades, had never been in jail, used no drugs, and only drank a little every now and then. She made friends easily and had a lot of them, though they seemed to cycle in and out of her life at a rather fast clip. She attended religious services with her family and was never a problem in that area either—although she didn't really live her creed, and she believed it even less. Mary Anne kept that to herself. No, she was not a problem child in the eyes of the adults in her life. Yet she did in fact have one enormous problem.

Mary Anne was a drama queen. Much as vampires are drawn to the dark, she thrived on gossip, backstabbing, betrayal, and good old-fashioned passive-aggressiveness with her peers. Her fangs, her tools of the trade if you will, were social media apps, especially Snapchat and Instagram. Her problem behavior was not constant; rather, it came in waves, depending, it seemed, on the state of her power reserves. When low she would flip on a friend or two by posting something glamorous about herself or something unflattering about others. In more honest moments, Mary Anne could admit, at least to herself, that she got a physical rush from this behavior, that it was thrilling. In the aftermath of tension within the coven, whoever might be in it at that moment, she felt absolutely sublime. It was truly intoxicating and deliciously so.

Aside from friends who chose to get off the merry-go-round, there was little in the way of tangible negative outcomes for Mary Anne. Everyone in the cone of mistrust seemed to enjoy the intensity of occasional tumult. To be sure, tears were shed and voices raised, but then came a restored pecking order, peppered with giggling. No "adults" knew any of this was happening, perhaps because young women don't often share such things with them, or perhaps because they weren't watching closely. At any rate, in their eyes Mary Anne was doing well in school and having the time of her life. And in some ways this was true. She had a full social calendar, and her friends enjoyed her company very much.

Until one of them didn't. This friend was raped. Mary Anne came to know her through their sorority, and it was at one of their events that the trauma occurred. She even knew something about the incident, or thought she did, by following posts and texts that sometimes go along with casual hookups. Mary Anne believed her friend was in search of this that night, and she also knew the guy she was with. The messages and pictures led her to think that her friend was very much a willing participant, and she did not believe the man involved was a rapist. The victim told a few of her friends, including Mary Anne, about what had happened, but did not specify what she'd consented to and what she had not. She was deeply ashamed of those details, but of course no one could know that. In short order, the usual flurry of posts and texts commenced, all begun by Mary Anne, though her friends would later weigh in, including, for a short time, the victim. She briefly tried to rectify the impression of her collusion but did not persist with this; it was like restraining an avalanche. Mary Anne in particular seemed to be on a campaign to ruin her friend's reputation in the sorority, though really that was not her purpose. Not directly anyway. Her true purpose was to consolidate power, and her friend's situation was only the most recent vehicle to accomplish this. But this time, and really for the first time in Mary Anne's life, this resulted in a disaster.

Her friend could bear the trauma of rape, and was actually well on her way to recovery in this regard. What she could not bear was the looming loss of her friends, of her friend group. She was called before their conduct review board and dismissed from a leadership role in the sorority. Suddenly, she found herself a pariah. Everyone went quiet with her, except, that is, for the reverberating rumor, which found its way back to her. Absolutely devastated, and with the extreme tunnel vision that accompanies such states, she hanged herself in her apartment. This was a tragedy of the highest order; and, as if the loss of a young and promising life, a bereft family, and grieving friends weren't enough, no one could truly understand what had taken place. Which means any healing would be incomplete. The usual memorials were observed, and counselors were brought in to assist, and though there was crying and kind words, the students themselves were otherwise stone cold silent.

Now Mary Anne experienced being flipped in the way she had practiced with others, except that this was the real deal, the real McCoy of searing rejections. She kept her status, technically speaking, in that she was not removed from any role she'd had before all this mess. She even continued to do well in class. But, like a silent, pernicious virus, the condemnation spread outward from her inner circle, first to her sorority, then to other friend groups. Everyone was seemingly polite—they still talked to her and included her in most things. What she lost was power, the kind of power that made others do emotional cartwheels for her over the most childish things. This came to a bitter, screeching halt. And there was not one thing Mary Anne could do about it, lest she implicate herself further. She felt the deepest panic she had ever felt, the kind of terror that gets into one's bones and is inexplicable, but there was no guilt. Not exactly. But it certainly visited her later.

Mary Anne confided in a rabbi on campus. Being a wise man, he confronted her in the most potent way possible but also urged her toward redemption. Among other things, he sent her to a campus therapist he'd worked with before, directing her to get right with God, others, and herself. When she told him that she'd gotten some Xanax from a campus physician, privately hoping this would somehow work and also get her off the hook with him, he roared with laughter. "Your disease is in the soul," he pronounced. "Stop playing games. Stop your bullshit. Starting now."

Not only did Mary Anne need to review why she was in college, she also needed to examine the purpose of her life. She had a gargantuan task ahead of her in somehow making amends alone. Hers was a crisis of meaning and ethics. This crisis emerged from the deepest of places within her, and no quick fix was possible. To her great fortune, her college not only provided adequate resources for such needs but also courageously set a tone for ethical conduct from her first moments as a student. (These two factors seem to go together in colleges.) Through her friends she experienced firsthand the consequences of various forms of malfeasance at college. She had always been able to escape consequences—until now. But with the college providing the necessary ingredients for her growth, there was hope for Mary Anne.

Co-opting Psychotherapy

College mental health work is a deeply rewarding profession. I feel privileged to walk alongside a young person and witness or assist his or her blooming into an authentic adulthood, facing fears and challenges along the way. I also feel blessed to have wonderful colleagues in student affairs who toil along with me. It is a joy to learn from them, and I like to think that I am able to assist them by interpreting and communicating the mental health needs of students and by offering a perspective that is incorporated into campus life.

But there are also frustrations, and here's one. On one hand, campus communities are now more educated and sensitive to students in need; faculty, staff, and parents routinely spot and refer a troubled student for counseling and other services. This is a good thing. Many students have obtained assistance in just this way. On the other hand, sometimes it is the third party that wants help for students, not the students themselves. When issues of safety are involved, this is not usually a problem; college mental health professionals are trained to find creative ways to provide help in such instances, up to and including the invocation of law relating to involuntary treatment.

The frustration emerges when the student's situation falls short of this safety mark—often far short. Disconcerting though it may be, students who, say, stare off into space in class may need help, but one cannot force it upon them. A student in grief over the loss of a family member is deserving of attention, but they do have the right to refuse it. The same is true about students who are homesick, partying too much, not doing well in class, angry at parents, not eating or sleeping well, sick of a roommate, and so on. Sometimes third parties, be they parents or university personnel, literally trip all over themselves trying to arrange for care, making multiple telephone calls, writing strings of emails, even visiting the campus counseling service, trying their best to shoehorn a student into treatment. Days and even weeks can pass while well-intentioned individuals engage in this frenetic activity. The labor involved here can really add up, for everyone. These actions are sometimes taken even when no one has asked the student if he would like help. There are even times, sadly and maddeningly, when someone resorts to trickery and coercion to get a student into therapy, such as posing as a student on the phone in order to set an appointment or threatening her with harsh consequences if she does not. Come on, people. This last scenario is a surefire way to make a student whom I don't even know hate me.

In quiet moments, which are few, counselors lean back and scratch their heads over these phenomena. Folks sure are anxious about something to resort to such behavior. From past experiences, counselors surmise that this anxiety may result from fear of being blamed if something goes wrong, for lack of clairvoyance in identifying a "potential shooter" (a reflection of the unfortunate times we live in), of facing the wrath of a powerful or "VIP" parent, or even a lack of skill in managing cheap, bullying behavior.

Not that counselors don't understand these anxieties. We do. These are all too human reactions in difficult circumstances. Sometimes we may be victim to them too. But let's all raise our game a bit. It is the student who needs to drive the therapy bus, not us. Short of life and death matters, often a problem needs to percolate for a while before someone feels motivated to get help. Humans, for the most part, don't take their hands off the stove until they feel some heat. We're just built that way, especially when we are young and not fully formed. It can be painful to watch a student twist in the wind before change happens, but this is a necessary stage many of us go through before transcending into maturity. In fact, we can contaminate the whole process by needling in it carelessly, thus blindly prolonging healing or enabling the continuation of disorder. I know in my heart no rational person wants this.

So, here's the deal. *Tell the student about your concern.* Encourage him to use the available resources. You can even be a benign pest by checking in with her repeatedly when you are really concerned. But, by all means communicate your respect for his autonomy and agency by giving him room to make his own choices and to be responsible for them. Also make sure that services and programs are oriented in this manner, especially those related to wellness. This course provides the fertilizer for students' continued growth, which is what we all want, including the students themselves.

David's mother sent multiple emails to the vice president, panic-stricken over her son's demeanor in the first few weeks of class. He had complained to her about not sleeping well, feeling anxious, missing a few classes. "I'm not sure I like it here," he said. Thus began many phone calls and texts back and forth, sometimes five or more per day. David himself was annoyed by this, though he certainly continued to complain to his mother. In her initial responses, the vice president tried to educate the mother about adjustment to college life and the resources available to David, which she dutifully passed along to him—and in which he had little interest, if you define not being willing to make a phone call as little interest. The mother's fervor only grew more intense when, during a call, David seemed lethargic and had not left his bed all day. He explained, "I've been watching videos all day." Nothing suggested he was in danger, but this was of no comfort to his mother. "You need counseling," she barked, loudly enough to get him to agree.

David's mother called the counseling service to get him an appointment but was told that David would have to call himself. She asked to speak with a counselor, who, through questioning, determined that there were no known signs of risk for harm to self or others and no history of mental health problems. He coached the mother on how best to continue working with David. She was urged to clearly communicate her expectations to him, especially about class attendance and grades, and to focus on expected outcomes rather than on fear of the unknown. The counselor could tell she was frustrated by this response, stating that she was a major donor to the school and that she knew the vice president personally, which she did not. It was actually another member of the family who knew him. The counselor remained calm and consistent, repeating suggestions and even explaining what to do in the event of an emergency.

So the mother's response was to call the vice president and blister the counseling service for being unhelpful. "They won't even see my son. I hope he doesn't kill himself while he waits for help." Partly trying to assist and partly in anxiety over the mother's stature, the vice president called the counseling manager and directed him to see the student that very day. The manager tried to explain, in generalities so as to protect David's privacy, that what the mother described does not happen in the counseling center. This did not appease the administrator, who understandably just wanted the situation "dealt with." The vice president asked the mother to come to campus at the end of the day and walk David into the center. In his urgent-visit paperwork, David denied being in a crisis of any kind and indicated that he did not really want to be there. But, as often happens, the counseling service saw him anyway.

David was not a minor, and he did not want his mother to attend the visit with him. They briefly argued over this in the lobby, but he had the law on his side. He was rightly angry over being manipulated into his first and brief exposure to psychotherapy. It was in these circumstances that David disclosed smoking marijuana throughout the day and having done so since early high school. "They are so clueless they never noticed," he added. Another daily habit was high-order gaming, involving dozens of others across the country. David was perfectly content with this lifestyle and said he planned to stay in school a while, and then tap his trust fund to move to California, "where people don't hassle you about this stuff." The counselor worked toward open communication about these things, but David refused to sign an authorization for this purpose. The counselor explained at length how communicating could actually improve things for him and his mother, but David was not interested. In this case, there were simple explanations for the noted patterns, but no one involved was willing to dialog in a useful or helpful manner.

Each participant acted on assumptions and rigidly held onto them. Such is the stuff that therapists often hear.

Even though she was offered a consulting relationship with another counselor in the center, the mother declined, punctuating the encounter with "We'll find someone else who will help us." She tried, but with the same outcome. In a subsequent meeting, the vice president articulated his frustration with "parents who find us unhelpful," exclaiming that "you counseling types think too much about confidentiality." Much, much later the manager of the counseling center told the vice president some composite narratives in an attempt to illustrate the ordinary pathology in family communication, but it seemed the moral of the story was lost. During their encounter, and fortunately for David, the counselor made this simple statement: "You know, I can help you have better relationships with your family, where each of you gets more of what you want." It seemed to fall flat at that time—as it often does; however, time passed and things changed.

David never did do well in school, and his parents divorced in a most grueling manner. His behavior did not change much, except that he matured some and learned to live his life in ways that did not alarm the people who cared for him. In particular, his feelings toward his parents softened a bit as he learned some details about their marital and financial stresses, including his father's affairs. Things got stormy for them all, but this time David was not so much at the center of it all.

A seed had been planted in that first therapy visit. David remembered what the counselor had told him and, perhaps more importantly, that she had protected his rights. He went back to see her, this time entirely on his own. The interpersonal "noise" having been removed from the question of his therapy, David was free to examine what he, and only he, thought was important. And so he did. They discussed issues related to his health, his responsibility to others, and just what he was escaping in the cloud of smoke and games. Considering what was happening at home, he had plenty to escape from. More than any of that, however, they worked on shoring up his personal boundaries and assertiveness skills, something that was sorely missing at home and which the school came close to unintentionally making worse. David learned that being honest doesn't mean sacrificing choice and freedom. And preserving a relationship in the midst of disagreement was an utterly novel concept for him. All the fuss that had happened came down to this plain truth.

A school must not contaminate its own growth processes. This is frighteningly easy to do, even for those with the best of intentions. It can happen, as it did in this illustration, through clumsy interpersonal functioning. It can also happen, even more frustratingly, through an entire system of responses—that is, through a paradigm and model of service. The intrapersonal paradigm in particular may fixate at the level of symptom, or problem behavior, and miss the why. For the why, we must inquire into David's developmental status and his entire context. Universities must have systems, that is to say, policies and procedures that promote this effort, or at least do not hobble it.

Lack of Faith in Experience

Much has been said and written on the subject of medication and its role in mental health care—perhaps too much—while comparatively little has been said or noticed about other ways the brain can be shaped to improve emotional well-being. Let's take a brief look at how experiences, both positive and negative, influence brain development and functioning.

A recent study, for example, examined the transmission of anxiety from parents to children (Budinger, Drazdowski, & Ginsburg, 2013). This research found that socially anxious parents imparted anxiety through specific parenting behaviors involving lack of warmth and affection, as well as criticism and doubt directed toward the child. The role of these experiences is thought to contribute to the development of anxiety apart from genetic contributions, because the latter alone are not thought to be sufficient in the etiology of an anxiety disorder. It does not require a tremendous leap to imagine that parental warmth and confidence provided to children reduces the likelihood of a future anxiety disorder. The experience of warmth and confidence is more powerful, in my opinion, and more lasting than any medication we might later give to the young adult to address his or her anxieties.

In another arena, a play-based method of teaching social interaction to autistic children, called ESDM, was shown to result in positive brain changes (Falco, 2012). Researchers studied brain activity in both autistic and nonautistic children, after the former had received the therapy for two years, and they could not identify apparent differences between the two groups. Clearly, this behavioral intervention altered brain activity in a desirable manner. I'll wager there are not many parents of children with autism who would not jump at the chance of trying this nonmedical, nonintrusive intervention; if only they could be given the chance, or that such behavioral interventions were as aggressively marketed as are medications.

Currently, one has to dig deep into the literature or perhaps be lucky enough to have an insightful and gifted care provider to access information about evidence-based psychological interventions. The American Psychological Association does maintain resources on these interventions on their very good website and Help Center (http://www.apa.org/helpcenter/index.aspx). I encourage consumers to be educated concerning these alternatives to physiological interventions, which, in my experience, are helpful at times and with some individuals, though the benefits come with a cost, are often illusory, and ultimately fade with time (Greenberg, 2016).

Experiences shape the brain. Those who have experienced stress, trauma, and deprivations have brains, and even appearances, that show this. Those who have experienced positive relationships and satisfaction of needs have brains that show that. It would seem, given that we know this, that individuals, groups, communities, and even countries would develop systems that promote the application of sound psychological principles to the advancement of human welfare. In our work with students, it is critical that we demonstrate faith in experience as an agent of change. Though one might say this is important for all people, it is crucial for those in their formative years: children, adolescents, and young adults. Promoting corrective experiences, while being persistent and patient in the process, is an enormously powerful method of brain and behavior change. It also falls precisely in the wheelhouse of higher education's mission.

Connie was an African American, first-generation college student. She was on the rise out of extreme poverty, her academic skills being her main ticket for this journey. She'd never had much difficulty in school. Some people thought the limitations of her primary schooling would hold her back, but she was, in fact, gifted. It just took a while for the right context to emerge so that others could witness it. Connie was very quiet and shy, and her communication skills further hid her talents, but this would later be revealed as resulting from lack of exposure and training, not lack of ability or intelligence. Once someone cared enough to show her, she was lightning quick on the uptake. Of course, this meant she would have to allow someone to get close enough to her to teach these softer skills, and this was in fact her biggest problem: Connie trusted no one, not even most of her family members.

In the early days of college, Connie's reticence was not much of a difficulty. She was busy getting core requirements out of the way, which she saw mostly as a necessary nuisance, and not particularly challenging. It was in her junior year that this changed, as her promising career was beginning to take shape. Due to her aloofness, a couple of her instructors believed that she would have difficulty acculturating into graduate school and the field of chemistry. One had attempted a conversation with her about this, but it did not go well. Connie became defensive and was irritated by him. She tended to be abrasive in such circumstances. But she was so talented, a diamond in the rough, that they decided to make her a special project, in the altruistic sense. Being white, they suspected their race would always be a hurdle, and mostly they were right; Connie needed every little erg of trust they could muster. They knew a black faculty member in sociology who seemed talented in the area of mentoring, so they approached him. He was delighted to help.

There was the matter of how to introduce the two without provoking Connie's defensiveness. Energetically, the prospective mentor offered: "She wants to go to grad school, right? Tell her to come to the Black Faculty and Staff Meeting. I'll be talking about graduate school in a couple of weeks." This was arranged, and the mentor ensured that another black faculty member, a female, was with him and involved. After the meeting they introduced themselves to Connie and told her about other functions she should attend to get used to academic life. She heard them, but was avoidant and did not respond for some time. Being experienced, the mentors knew how to follow up. They sent her frequent emails about events of the BFSA and its membership. They called her, too, gradually intensifying their invitations and couching them in the context of being professionally successful. "We've been through this, and we know," they would plead. At times Connie was annoyed by their intrusions into her quiet world, but she also knew they spoke the truth and that she might benefit from their wisdom, or at least their connections.

Besides, her chemistry advisor also encouraged her to stay in touch with them.

So finally it happened that she attended a meal at the home of a BFSA member where the mentors were present. It was as pleasant as these things could be for her. There were introductions all around and a few discussions about professional fields, campus politics, and the like. Connie absorbed it all thirstily. But she only nibbled at the delicious food, and this was noticed by the female mentor. Later, she pulled Connie aside and asked how she was doing, noting that she looked thin, fatigued, and wan. "To be a good chemist you have to take care of yourself, girl," she said. In this way, the mentors learned that Connie was not eating much and had problems sleeping. They suggested she get a check-up, and she did so. There too she was told she was underweight and also screened for depression, and offered an antidepressant, which she refused. Soon thereafter, Connie got into a heated argument with an instructor, during which she cursed, "You're too fucking pushy." She then was required to meet with the dean, who issued a stern warning about such behavior and tried to determine what more might be bothering her. Connie tearfully relented, "I'm just so tired. I just want to sleep but I can't." The dean told her she must do something about this, and he offered several referrals, but these too were refused. Persisting, the dean learned about the mentors and arranged a meeting with them. There was now some important, purely interpersonal leverage in working with Connie, and this paved the way for helping her turn things around.

The mentors learned that Connie struggled with overcoming deprivation, not so much because she didn't know what to do for herself, or even that she couldn't—scholarship money made it more than possible for her to take care of the basics. No, this was a psychological issue. She had learned a pattern of sacrifice early in life, and she felt guilty when she had something her family did not. This was so deeply ingrained in her that she robotically sent her last penny home, instead of buying food or other comforts. In addition to normal academic stress, her anxiety about relationships and poor diet were the cause of her insomnia. The mentors spotted a problem with nurturance, in no small part because they too had experienced this at one time. With the fervor that can only come from transcendence, which they had both achieved, the mentors forcefully and empathically confronted Connie about her responsibility to herself. "If you're not careful you won't be of any use to anybody. You have to have milk in the breast to feed a baby, don't you? How are you going to do that if you ain't got no milk?!" They all cried together, from the most powerful place of shared experience and stark truth.

The mentors managed to get Connie to agree to eat a meal with either or both of them at least once a day. This idea sputtered at first, but it gradually took hold of Connie. During these meals, they laughed, and Connie was praised for her gifts and successes along the way. They counseled her on the finer skills needed in academia, as each presented itself naturally in her coursework and other activities. Without fully realizing it, Connie was being nurtured and, more importantly, learning how to accept this help. It was this acceptance that helped her learn to trust. One way the mentors won this trust was to help her sort out her finances and learn how she could reasonably help her family while also taking care of her basic needs. Everything about her improved: her diet, her sleep, her appearance, and her academic vitality. Her brain being nurtured and calmed, Connie was transformed by two gifted helpers.

Experience shapes the brain. Paradigms and systems that promote all avenues of change provide for transformational experiences like Connie's. Her change was neither quick nor efficient. It took time and unique points of view, which, to her good fortune, were part of her college experience. One could say that it was pure happenstance in her case, but it need not be. Flexible, inclusive, and comprehensive helping systems can and do provide for alternative approaches that most students need.

Fear-Based Responding

In our current age, stimulated by tragedies such as the killings at Virginia Tech, the collective campus antennas are at peak height. Neuronal receptors fire rapidly at even the faintest indication of crises. On the one hand, this increased sensitivity was needed. Law books record that many a sleepy school missed warning signs in the past. This atmosphere has made mental health sexy! We're in demand, and folks want us everywhere, through our consultation and outreach services. This is what I dreamed about early in my career, when we all felt like John the Baptist hollering in the wilderness.

Talk about answered prayers! The other hand of this situation, the shadow of sensitivity, is a kind of hyperreactive responding to student distress. Once, in a consultation with a faculty member, it was suggested that a student was a "shooter," and the sole piece of objective evidence offered was that the student had a Mohawk hair style. This gives new meaning to the adage "going off half-cocked." In another scenario, a mother demanded to sit in on every therapy session and record them with her cell phone, ostensibly to monitor her adult child's every move. While acute awareness is positive, overreactions can result in the very things we are trying to avoid: students seeing help as punitive, intolerance for diversity and eccentricity (and therefore individuality), and a constraining lack of faith in our youth and their maturation process. Worse yet, students caught in this whirlwind may come to believe they are dangerous and come to act accordingly—"because they think I am this way anyway."

Popular media accounts contain tales of distressed students who were medicated, hospitalized, suspended, or withdrawn from enrollment, many times apparently with haste and therefore before anyone could understand the entire context and its embedded developmental crisis. Consider a female who is by all accounts manic and aggressive, dabbling in mood-altering substances, but who, after enough time to be thorough, is found to be legitimately in a rage over trauma—trauma that she is not ready to expose and, even if she were, is unable to articulate in language. In such a case as this, fear-based responding will damage her further, partly by prematurely identifying her as "sick" when the true illness lies elsewhere.

Mark was raised in a Pentecostal family that observed strict rules of comportment, especially in the area of dress and romantic relationships. All through high school, he was expected to wear black slacks and a white buttoned and collared shirt. Dating of any kind was forbidden until he was 20. Mark lived much of his life in a state of looming threat, of his father's religious rages, of condemnation, and of what he learned about a harsh and punitive God. For many years, others would have noted his obedience but not the anxiety he carried with him at all times. He was in a kind of stasis in this tension, until the forces of puberty arrived and intensified his predicament. In part because this awakening was all around him in his peers, and in part because it was already in him, Mark would ruminate about girls, school dances, field parties arranged by students in the county, and other things that teenagers do. For him these were taboo—which drastically increased their appeal, as well as the level of psychic turmoil with which he had to wrestle.

It was in this context that Mark arrived at college. In the beginning, given that college was a novel stressor, he returned to previous levels of functioning in the form of obedience and the "right" conduct. He dutifully fulfilled his academic requirements, checking each one off like one might do in a factory assembly line. In other words, there was no emotion, no motivation supporting the enterprise. As he was commanded, Mark phoned home and provided a daily report on his activities, hour by hour. "You are living as God commands us" was the only fatherly acknowledgment he received at the end of these mind-numbing status reports. At college, Mark never heard from his mother unless he asked his father if he could speak to her, which was agreed to, albeit somewhat reluctantly by his father.

At first Mark was disgusted by many things he saw in the residence hall. He found the alcohol abuse and general debauchery to be genuinely repulsive. He'd never seen blatant female sexuality before, that is to say, flirting, innuendo, and provocative dress, and this both appalled and aroused him. He overheard tales of sexual encounters told by his male floor mates but could not have known what the rest of us do: that these are mostly made of hubris and embellishment and downright deceit. To him they represented the fallen, the sewer of humanity, and those who will be condemned and never see God's face. He was also incredibly excited by the thoughts and images produced in him by such stories. Due to the amount of suppression involved, along with the volume of exposure to various forms of sexuality, Mark was walking a very high psychic tightrope, and sooner or later the strain would cause the rope to snap. His first two years of school were marked by this high-wire act, with no resolution in sight.

But then, as is inevitable, Mark turned 20 and in short time met Abby, who attended the same campus church. She ostensibly held the same beliefs as he did, but these were already transforming for her, which made her far more rebellious within the Pentecostal faith anyway. After securing the requisite parental permissions, Mark and Abby went on his very first date. Taking an enormous risk, he dressed in jeans and a green polo shirt. The jeans may have been scandalous, but the shirt had the school logo, so it seemed passable to him. The coffee shop date would have been unremarkable were it not that Mark had no earthly idea how to talk with a woman. Honestly, he did not know how to talk with any peer; he was only comfortable with male authority figures. What conversation they attempted was awkward. There were furtive attempts to talk about church, their family and homes, and that was about it. After the snack and coffee it was over, and he took Abby home. At her door, Mark leaned in to kiss her cheek, but she recoiled and laughed. Though she was simply nervous, Mark was enraged and yelled that she would be cursed for treating him this way. Abby attempted an apology and explanation, but Mark had already wheeled around and left.

He did not sleep for two days. Mark was totally unprepared for this event, having been taught that women should be submissive to God and men, and that's all he had ever seen, in church relationships and at home. There was no solace in his faith, only wrath. So when he consulted religious texts for direction, it was wrath that he found. Mark began a barrage of texts and other messages to Abby, berating her for her disobedience to God and warning her of a "correction" that was to come. He persisted through her demands that he stop, continuing daily messages and even delivering a note to her home. His language included examples of various bloodbaths in his Bible, waged on those who had gone astray. Mark never threatened Abby directly, but his assault was hardly comforting to her, and she was afraid.

Thus Mark came to the attention of the dean of students and campus law enforcement. As his father had told him, his faith would be tested, and he must "continue the good fight." Mark continued in his campaign after stern warnings had been issued. By then, Abby's family was involved, and with their encouragement Abby filed a formal conduct complaint against him. This set off a number of meetings and hearings, including an interview with the police, which was voluntary and to which he agreed. In these encounters Mark centered his responses on biblical passages and concepts and did not waver from his sense of righteousness and indignation. Various personnel thought him possibly delusional and dangerous. He was found responsible and prohibited from having contact with Abby. They also wanted to refer him for counseling, but this service was contracted out and did not cover mandated referrals. Her parents demanded that he be expelled. Even so, Mark was resolved in his faith, and his communications with Abby continued. The school, concerned for Abby's safety, did not mount any other type of effort to address Mark's issues because there weren't any more resources they could think of. He was suspended.

No doubt anyone would find Mark's behavior troubling. That the school had to respond is also understandable. But resorting to one avenue of intervention, in this case escalating restrictions to academic status, simply due to a lack of foresight, is highly problematic. It is dangerous to upset a fragile student's psychic balancing act merely because it is not understood or is, more to the point, confused with dangerousness. Doing so can lead to the very outcomes we are working to prevent. In reality, Mark never posed a physical threat to anyone. He never characterized himself as the actor in violent revenge; he only used biblical metaphors.

Furthermore, his rage was not so much about Abby as it was about his basic needs being thwarted, by the suppression imposed on him by his father and his own beliefs. An astute therapist or clergy person could have arrived at this assessment, had these been available and incorporated into response protocols. In that case, other avenues of response could have been developed, allowing for an appropriate response to inappropriate behavior but also giving Mark a positive framework within which to grow. Overly rigid responses and systems usually do not provide this degree of sophistication in the management of troubling behavior, and they often unintentionally facilitate its continuation, through motivation by fear. With his suspension, Mark is actually *more* likely to act out again, possibly with Abby, because he was not given another viable way to bring his feelings to resolution.

A Review of Ethics in Matters of Orientation

It does not take a well-trained ethicist to spot the paradigmatic problems noted previously, but it helps to review general ethical principles as they pertain to dynamics in various philosophical orientations. In all codes for mental health professionals, the notion of *advancing human welfare* is of primary importance and is grounded in a spirit of caring and compassion. Since the adoption of any paradigm or model involves choices of perspective, therefore potentially abandoning or rejecting others, we may start off with a limited point of view of humans and their suffering. It is within these limitations that ethical problems arise, because, by definition, helpers will limit what they see in and do for students and clients. It is, therefore, essential for IHEs to be thorough and comprehensive in their selection of paradigms and models for mental health service delivery. There is an ethical imperative to do so, as that posture is what may best lead to the promotion of human welfare in its fullest sense.

All mental health professionals are also instructed to do no harm. An ill-fitting paradigm or service model, mismatched to the needs of the local community, may do just the opposite, in spite of the best intentions of its leaders. Psychologists in particular are given this warning: "Because psychologists' scientific and professional judgments and actions may affect the lives of others, they are alert to and guard against personal, financial, social, organizational, or political factors that might lead to misuse of their influence" (APA, 2017). Note the use of the terms *organizational* and *political*. The process of making choices in paradigm and service model is highly representative of both, even—and perhaps especially—when done by fiat. There is no escaping ethical reality and responsibility in such a process. It is incumbent upon all helpers to address these issues in any way they can in order to advance human welfare and prevent or limit harm.

Helpers are also obliged to establish *relationships of trust* with those with whom they work, and to be faithful in that work. This implies a basis in *truthfulness* in our communications and behavior. We must manage conflicts of interest well, and these are inherent in the rough and tumble world of competing political and economic objectives. Still, we function in this world to ensure the just and fair involvement of all for the betterment of those we serve. To that end, helpers are concerned with the ethical behavior of everyone involved, not just themselves. The decisions that administrators make, and their reasons for making them, are therefore relevant to this obligation. When decisions about paradigms are made in haste, in laziness, or in deference to guild politics and economics, the risk for broken trust and dishonesty is exceedingly high. It takes the faithful attention of all to avoid failure in the pursuit of these ethical commitments.

There is the imperative of *seeking justice* for all persons. Every community includes persons who are being deprived of justice in some way, large or small. In all our work, helpers must address this unfairness, which many times originates at the level of system, policy, and orientation toward the learner and those who fund their pursuits. Justice is what makes choices in paradigm and service model so critical. Extreme care ought to be taken in this process, but all too often it is not. The pursuit of justice incorporates *respect for privacy, autonomy and self-determination, and culture*. Sometimes, in the construction of a service model, one or more of these forms of respect may be unintentionally impaired, particularly when attention, and therefore allegiance, is directed toward the funding model. That we may have to provide for funding, thereby serving two masters, does not mean that we must wholly subjugate one to the other.

In short, those working within all paradigms and models for responding offices should have well-tuned antennas but also be imbued with enough time, patience, and human service skill to identify both student need and risk and their underlying psychic architecture, *which is always present*. It is not good enough to focus only on risk. It is not good enough to focus only on funding. When a college is off the mark, it may well fuel a student's developmental crisis, lengthening its time to resolution and quite possibly creating other points of stagnation or trajectories for students. This type of responding, by individuals and by systems, results in both ethical lapses and repetitive loops of problems administrators have to address. To limit or redirect reflexive responses, mental health professionals should be highly involved in discussions about paradigm and service model. Even after that, helpers ought to be put into the service of training the campus community to respond competently to student risk and need. This is precisely the role of a superior and comprehensive counseling center.

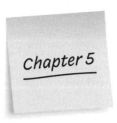

Chapter 5

Outreach and Consultative Work at College Counseling Centers

College counseling centers experience identity crises for many reasons, often not because of confusion within the center itself. Many centers have a clear mission and vision, and their staff members are focused on and diligent about the services they offer, especially in those centers that are accredited by the International Association of Counseling Services, Inc. (IACS). At the same time, some centers may demonstrate paradigmatic conflict as they wrestle with seamless linking of services representing the four paradigms or, more likely, multiple service models. When a service is constructed in a thoughtless or haphazard manner, without attention to paradigm and model, there will be confusion. Frontline staff members are there to do the work we ask of them: psychotherapy, outreach programming, consultative services, and in many cases, training. Their hands are full; they simply do not have time to hack through a thicket of philosophical conflict.

That is the job of administrators. It is they who should devote time to erecting seamless linkages among paradigms and models so that staff members have an unambiguous road map for their work. Though confusion can appear anywhere in a center's slate of services, nowhere is this more obvious than in its outreach and consultative work. First and foremost, many campus stakeholders are not aware that such services exist, and when they are, many are not knowledgeable about them. This ignorance causes one level of problems with the center's identity. Some centers may do very little if any outreach work and may only provide consultations within the host department itself. These centers could not be IACS-accredited without changes, and they are often quite isolated from the campus community and seen by its members as a "dark and mysterious place where they do counseling." In other cases, these services are provided but mainly from within the intrapersonal paradigm, while the service purports adherence to an extrapersonal or other paradigm, or vice versa. This inattentive mixing causes another level of identity problem: organizational dissociation or mission creep.

Definitions

Since some of the issues begin with definitional problems, let us start there. I offer the following:

- Outreach services are oriented toward prevention or education and involve the preplanned, structured delivery of mental health expertise to two or more people, usually in person and outside the center, and usually in the format of presentations, group discussions, displays, events, and literature.

- Consultative services involve the unplanned, unstructured delivery of mental health expertise to at least one person, often about another person of concern, usually inside the center and often over the telephone, and usually in a quasi-confidential format. (I say *quasi* here because a formal, written agreement to provide confidentiality may or may not be offered.)

These are certainly not the only definitions. IACS (2016) defines outreach as "preventive programming focused on the developmental needs of students, to maximize the potential to benefit from their academic experience" (Standard II.C.), and consultation as "training and professional development to members of the university community, to foster an environment that is beneficial to the intellectual, emotional, and physical development of students" (Standard II.D.). Those within an intrapersonal paradigm, primarily medically oriented services, may define outreach as "public health," framed by disease concepts, and define consultation as an adjunct service provided at the direction of a provider and possibly directly only to him or her. Beyond accreditation requirements, a center may define these services, and limit their scope, in any way its leaders wish. Philosophical confusion is a much greater risk when accreditation does not exist or is not a goal, or when the accreditation does not fully address or support outreach and consultative work performed directly by mental health professionals.

Purpose and Goals of Outreach and Consultative Services

The purpose of outreach and consultative services is to educate and prepare the IHE community to respond effectively to students and their mental health needs. Central to this purpose is the notion of *competence*. IHEs seek, among other things, to produce competent students and, ultimately, citizens of the world. Everyone is aware how this competency is achieved in the classroom. Fewer are aware that such competency is also achieved outside the classroom—perhaps even most of it, given the amounts of time spent in each area. Such is the mission of most divisions of student affairs or student life. But if IHEs are to deliver the skills necessary to attain competence, the staff involved must be competent in providing it. Mental health services and professionals not only possess content but also process knowledge concerning the emotional well-being of students; that is, not only the *what* of mental health but also the *how*. These professionals can help individuals, groups, and communities interpret patterns of student thought, feeling, and behavior, as well as determine how these may be addressed competently and effectively. This truth is what makes campus mental health service outreach and consultative work essential. It is also *why* it is given deserved attention by IACS.

For centers and staff members to perform well, they must be competent themselves, and this is achieved through training and continuing education. This training is mainly focused, however, on micro-level skills, rarely on paradigmatic perspectives. Without proper orientation to paradigm, micro-level skills may represent a hodgepodge of conflicting perspectives, which in turn may limit or reduce one's ability to inculcate competence in the community. Consider an example:

A campus has observed a marked increase in assertiveness problems and aggressive behavior in one residence hall, though historically it has happened in other locations as well. The counseling service offers outreach, and the housing staff is aware of its availability. They contact the center for programming to help them address the issues, which they describe, and a program is scheduled and developed. As a portion of the problem appears to relate to the disordered behavior of one or two students, the presentation and subsequent consultations with housing staff focus on mental illness—what it is and how it may be managed (an intrapersonal perspective). The staff find the service somewhat helpful because it did speak to an aspect of the problem. The pattern continues, however, and the staff feel something has been left undone.

What remains undone? The answer involves elements of the extrapersonal, societal, and perhaps spiritual-existential paradigms. Even other elements of the intrapersonal paradigm were not included, such as a perspective on current trends in the development of young adults having to do with interpersonal skills and emotional intelligence. It is not uncommon for today's students to "cocoon" in their fully wired room with private bathroom, streaming videos or gaming. As today's students are digital natives, this pattern is not new to them; it was their pattern at home too. Thus many students have interpersonal deficits, too much isolation, and too few hours off the screen and in the presence of another person. While attention to one or two students in need may be relevant for those individuals, it will not be for the rest of the community, which needs help to reduce the cocooning, maximize interaction, and develop the soft skills that empower good mental health and are sought by employers today. Conflict management, assertiveness training, role-playing and rehearsal, ethics education, and group processing activities may all be useful in this scenario, as these are reflected in other paradigms and models.

The possibilities for the foci of outreach programming are nearly limitless. This programming may cover any aspect of human thought, feeling, and behavior that pertains to well-being, academic success, and community involvement. Ideally, it is targeted to the IHE's self-assessment, described previously. Every campus has its own unique pattern of strengths and areas for improvement, so the outreach menu ought to reflect that pattern in its content and delivery. Mental health professionals are best suited to construct, deliver, and evaluate this programming, in no small part owing to their skill level in managing interpersonal relationships with stakeholders and collaborators.

Another reason mental health professionals are best suited for this work relates to the goal of *interpreting the developmental picture* of students for administrators and others. Much young adult behavior can be alarming or confusing, and most laypersons are somewhat at a loss how best to respond. Faculty and staff are not infrequently confronted by disruptive or antagonistic behavior, threatening or belligerent language, hyperkinesis or lethargy, and explorations into identity that raise eyebrows. Sometimes these behaviors indicate mental illness; most of the time they do not. Mental health professionals can determine the difference and train community members to assist in that determination and also to help staff not to underrespond or overrespond to students. This determination and response is crucial; it can set the student on a path toward growth or it can derail his or her development significantly. For this reason, college counseling centers, particularly those with a developmental and extrapersonal orientation, are able to impart a sense of patience and faith in the young adult. Nearly all students, particularly those in difficult contexts, will experience emotional volatility, and it will not be neatly contained in their living spaces. When campus partners contain or absorb the energy, not reacting as though every signal originates from an intrapersonal source, they remain open to what may emerge as a positive developmental trajectory, or a contextual fix, and the student remains free to grow. Too, and perhaps more importantly, the student does not erect an identity of a self that is defective, disfigured, or ill. *That conception may well last a lifetime.* Here is but one example.

Bev has been described as manic and dangerously thin, but really what has gotten everyone's attention is her anger. She has blurted profanities in class and used vaguely threatening language, mainly to the males in her residence. Her grades are slipping. Many of those around her, in and out of class, are uncomfortable and anxious, though no one has been specifically targeted. Following the usual procedures, she has come to the attention of a behavior intervention team, and a referral to the mental health service has been initiated but declined. She lands in another provider's office, is diagnosed with bipolar disorder and medicated accordingly, all after about 30 minutes of interaction. The relief of those involved is palpable.

But the success of the intervention is an illusion. The urgency of the matter has translated into haste; no one has slowed down long enough and given Bev the time she needs to tell her story. (And there is *always* a story.) Because she is communicating through behavior and not language, Bev can be assumed to have reasons for her inarticulate expressions. After a few months of equivocal progress, Bev finally goes to the counseling service. In the hands of a skilled therapist who gives her plenty of time, the truth is learned. Bev is righteously angry. She reveals a history of various forms of abuse in both the distant and the recent past. It has been my experience that most people have very good reasons for their behavior, no matter how alarming, bizarre, or self-defeating it may be. Once time and good listening is applied generously, such students have an opportunity to correct the course and head off in the direction of hope and success.

Incidentally, this scenario reveals inherent limitations of the intrapersonal paradigm in that individuals may actually "meet the criteria" for diagnosis but in essence not actually "have" that disorder, which does not compute in some systems. What they "have" is a dis-order created by a combination of contextual, developmental, and communicative factors. Systems and paradigms in IHEs simply must have the capacity to detect and work with such individuals. This example and many others like it highlight the critical nature of interpretation of human behavior. Differing interpretations emerge, depending on the training and background of the interpreter and, perhaps more importantly, the paradigm and service model from which they operate. The philosophical compass is what will orient the IHE ship, and it should be set according to the culture and needs of the institution and its students.

The Appreciation of Training

We come again to the necessity of training by mental health professionals. Because of identity issues affecting many centers, campus leaders often fail to see the center as the crucial training resource it rightly ought to be. Enlightened administrators will see a clear connection between the behavioral issues they manage, the skills repertoire of the counseling staff, and the philosophical orientation toward persons and their problems in living, all of which should be in synch and match the IHE's needs. When this connection is established in their minds, they become champions of outreach and consultation conducted by the counseling service. This type of leadership is imperative for the thriving and successful counseling center. Mental health professionals and managers do not generally receive any training in marketing or even business acumen. They possess clinical and interpersonal skills but need assistance to impact the entire campus community at maximum levels. Upper administration hopefully sees this need and works to infuse the center into wider and wider social circles on campus so that it may fully manifest the gifts it has. This act of appreciation and linking, while routine for the skilled upper administrator, is the breath of life for a successful and impactful counseling center.

Effective Campus Consultations

In the college counseling world, consultation refers to delivering mental health expertise to concerned third parties, such as faculty, staff, parents, and other community members. On most campuses, the community sees the counseling service as a valuable resource, one that offers all its members some assistance in helping students effectively.

This aspect of services is rife with both potential conflict and opportunity. On the one hand, the student is always the focus of services and often also the client; on the other hand, the institution is also always the client—the corporate client. There are a few times when the needs of each are in conflict. I submit, however, that such occasions are rare. Mostly, there is enormous overlap among the needs of the two. Indeed, the IHE and the

student each actually wants the same thing: to retain and graduate young adults. My direct experience has been that when there
is conflict, it's often because one or both are nurturing needs
that are unreasonable, though that is of course open to debate.

So here, then, in no particular order, are a few tips on delivering effective consultations on campus.

*Establish the identification of the primary client, and do it early
and often.* If the student about whom someone is concerned is
a client of the center, she is the primary client, and the obligations to her are paramount. In this case, the institution becomes
a secondary client, though in this context this does not mean its
needs are inferior, only that they must be addressed by someone
who does not have a dual role with the student, unless the student has authorized such activity. The consultant also needs to
have maximum objectivity concerning the organizational con-
sultee, which is more difficult to achieve when there is a direct
relationship with the student.

Respond promptly, every time. The fortunes of college counseling rest on our showing up—always. It is often expensive to
do so, considering the labor involved, but there is a huge return
on investment. Don't just say no; find a way to help and tell the
other stakeholders that you will do so. Successful businesses
put the consumer first. There is no reason why we should not do
this as well. Even when needs conflict or dual roles exist, there is
always a way to be helpful. It may take some time and creativity
to pull this off, so one could always say "I'm not sure how to help
you, but keep talking to me and I will find a way."

Establish and maintain clear boundaries and expectations. Some
requests are appropriate, but some clearly are not; for example,
when someone asks for privileged information for which there is
no authorization, or if there is no risk for harm to self or others.
You could be the FBI or a parent or an administrator. It does not
matter. Abrogating the therapy relationship in this way can be
fatal to therapy, now and perhaps well into the future for a student. That's a really bad thing. At the same time, there may be

a need driving the request which can in fact be satisfied. Figure out what that need is.

Keep your word and be consistent. Whatever happens, do what you say you will do and do it every time. Since we're all human here, we make mistakes, and no one can rightly tell you that you can't. But if you do, own up to it and set it right whenever possible.

Consultations are wonderful opportunities to get things back on a good path, for the student as well as the community. Often the circumstances behind the consultation represent the logical though negative conclusion of unhealthy relating and thwarted expectations that have festered for quite some time. It is a kind of bubble that needs to burst, but all involved sometimes prevent or avoid that from happening because it is an uncomfortable, awkward, or painful process. An effective consultation facilitates the bursting in a controlled manner, so that maximum learning and change can occur—which is exactly what everyone needs, whether they know and want it or not.

Seemingly out of nowhere, Barb came to the attention of residence hall and dean of students' staff due to reports of apparently suicidal statements. Floor mates had repeatedly overheard her saying things like "I can't live this way anymore" and "This has got to end" over the course of her sophomore year. At first, bystanders took these as the all-too-common signs of stress, because so many students talk this way at times. But with Barb there was something foreboding in her facial expressions and mannerisms that increasingly worried the witnesses. She was otherwise a quiet and retiring student, never calling attention to herself in any way, so her behavior was perplexing to everyone involved.

She dutifully met with staff members but was reticent and volunteered no clarifying information beyond saying "You don't have to worry, I am not going to kill myself." Her delivery was not reassuring, however, so the assistant dean of students referred her to the counseling center for an evaluation. Barb gave the appearance of demurring but in fact participated in the call to set an appointment there, and she subsequently attended the appointment. In the meantime, her roommates' parents began pressuring residence hall staff to relocate Barb to another room. A hall director contacted the counseling service, seeking advice about the severity of Barb's problems and an opinion about relocating her. The counselor who fielded this call took down the information and questions, explaining that a fuller response would be forthcoming, and passed this information along to Barb's counselor. In her initial visit, Barb's counselor had already conducted a routine risk assessment and obtained authorizations for him to speak with both housing and dean of students staff members. Beyond appearing depressed and very frustrated, Barb had not offered much of an explanation to the counselor either, other than a brief and cryptic reference to conflicts with her father.

The counselor followed up with the referring staff member and explained that he judged Barb to be at very low acute risk to harm herself and at no known risk to harm anyone else. In keeping with the ethics of administrative neutrality, which advises against the dual role of being both a therapist and a person who engages in administrative actions on a student, he could not speak directly to relocating her. He could, however, offer recommendations about helpful responses to Barb, which he did. "She needs all the support we can provide to her. It would be a bad idea to add losses of any kind." The hall director then encouraged the roommates to remain in dialog with Barb, working out their concerns together. She offered to assist in this conversation. One of the three roommates instead chose to relocate herself, largely at the overreactive urging of her own parents and not out of any real fear of her own.

In one of her therapy visits Barb expressed frustration at not being able to register for the following academic term. "They want me to pay my account down first," she said. In her intake paperwork Barb had indicated that two scholarships were funding her education, and the counselor remembered this. He asked what had become of her scholarship money. The question was met with silence at first, Barb's face gradually turning ashen and knotted with worry. "What's really going on, Barb?" Still, she did not answer. The counselor ended that visit by telling Barb that, working together, they could certainly sort out the problem, but only if she told the truth. This work would continue in future visits.

Barb then happened to see her departed roommate on campus, and let loose a barrage of insults for abandoning her. As she had done before, the roommate alerted her parents, who then took matters to the campus police, demanding that Barb be expelled. "She can't study in this situation, thinking that the girl is going to hurt her. This is ridiculous!" they bellowed. Thus started another flurry of calls to the counseling center, this time by an officer addressing the public safety aspects of this problem. The counselor arranged to have Barb come in for a crisis visit right away and again was able to speak with the officer. First, he confronted Barb's poor decision and added, "You must work on your issues directly, by telling me what is happening to your money. If you keep on in this way, you will dig a deeper hole with this college and maybe sabotage your own education." He repeated his earlier opinion and recommendation to the officer, who finalized this process with a notification to the student conduct office.

During another visit, Barb relented, and told a painful story about her father's drug addictions and his harassment, including following her around on campus at unexpected times. "He doesn't care about me. He just wants my money." The counselor gambled and asked "How does he get it?" Barb then revealed a history of his pressuring her to send him money, and later accessing her accounts by stealing her passwords. Throughout this ordeal he threatened that he would not let her keep her car or talk to or see her younger brother if she didn't help him. For several visits they worked through aspects of this experience, empowering her to stop the abuse. This work was very frightening to Barb, but she came to trust her counselor, a male who demonstrated the needed respect and honesty.

She was walked through the needed resources on campus, involving the security of her identity, financial protections, legal recourse, and her personal safety. This required a massive volley of consultations by the counselor with multiple campus offices, explaining the full context of her situation. Barb was given a new student identification number, and she entered new passwords, to which only she had access, due to a new mailing address and other features. Her father initially escalated his harassment, but this time the police intervened, and he was removed from the campus. Gradually Barb's situation improved, though the therapy work of dealing with family dynamics continued for some time.

In Barb's case we see a complex problem that was addressed partly by therapy but largely by a supportive community response, triggered by sophisticated consultation. The counselor and other staff had to withstand other, compelling pressures, including any urges to blame the victim and remove the perceived threat. Only through patience and gathering information were those outcomes, very damaging to a traumatized student, averted. Very often the best consultations involve a degree of faith in the young adult in moments when this is precisely the most difficult thought or emotion to register and act upon. The well-trained and equipped college mental health professional is often just the right person to engage in this process.

Developing Community Responsiveness

Conkin (2000) articulated all that was lost as we moved out of villages, particularly for Americans. He implied that human beings were not really "designed" to live in an area any larger than a village. This type of community, it could be argued, afforded us the greatest opportunity for both advancement and mutual protection. This point of view is also appropriate as we consider how best to manage the mental health of students (and ourselves). We certainly seem to do better when we are looking out for and helping each other, just as villagers often did in days past.

College environments are inherently protective, due largely to proximity to others, availability of supportive resources, and the possibility of protective monitoring offered by some offices, such as a dean of students or the campus police. At the same time, college campuses can be very large and, depending on housing features and a student's choices, isolating. Here is where "the village" comes into play.

It takes an entire campus community, the village, to advance and protect students. Too often this responsibility is left solely to certain supportive offices, such as a counseling center. While such services can and do work wonders, going a long way toward the preservation of mental health, they simply cannot and never will be able to accomplish it alone. Just as villagers must cooperate to survive, so all campus constituencies must work together for the sake of its members. Effective consultation services can assist in this "working together," partly by centering the change targets on solid interpretations of behavioral patterns. Everyone has a role and no one should be excused from this duty. From salaried administrators to those on hourly wages, each community member has knowledge of and is witness to issues students face, no matter how remote they may seem. The primary task is to sensitize everyone to this fact, and to give them the tools they need to communicate accordingly. It is the simple buddy system, which has stood the test of time since we all lived in caves, and it still works today.

The single best antidote to a host of emotional health issues and social ills is the proactive involvement of the entire campus community. When we all care for one another and are paying attention, we can resolve seemingly insurmountable problems. We can prevent episodes of depression. We can reduce anxieties and stress. We can prevent suicide. This attentiveness is absolutely necessary as each campus has its own unique set of "pathogens," forces that, perhaps unintentionally, create negative psychological states. Here are a few examples:

- The "party town"
- Fierce academic competitiveness
- Fixations and fears about image and status
- Preference for the privileged
- The bohemian village
- Urbanity or rurality
- Spiritual purity

Focusing on the individual alone is never good enough. We must also see individuals in their many contexts, including the result of any psycho-pathogenic elements of campus culture. That in place, we can then reach out to educate and prepare the village. The training for this approach is available on most campuses. The skills needed are elementary and easy for community members to learn. Often, what stands in the way is the attitude that "this is not my job," sometimes borne of an inaccurate assessment of liability. Training can address such myths as well. When you boil it all down, all that is needed is a street-level human response to student concerns. Once others have been notified, more sophisticated interventions can be arranged and matters put into capable hands. The work is not difficult to do and, just like CPR, everyone can and should be familiar with it.

Preparing the university community to respond to mental health needs ought to be required training on every college campus. And if you really want to develop this skill worldwide, incorporate it into all early education.

Kathleen belonged to a tightly knit community of LGBTQ students and a student organization called the Rainbow. Though the school they attended was in a town considered politically moderate, perhaps some distance left of center, most of its students came from very conservative areas, and occasionally conservative pressures were brought to bear on the small college. And so it happened when a gubernatorial election led to the emergence of a "red state," or the dominance of the conservative political party. During his successful campaign, the governor made statements about fragile college students being indoctrinated with Marxist philosophies and given shelter in which they are "encouraged to be twisted." "This will come to an end," he howled. Then, in the rallies that followed, crowds chanted white power slogans and carried "Throw Them Out!" signs, listing many undesirable groups—"brown people," "foreigners," "the gays." To students, the message was clear and a source of great anxiety. Kathleen in particular was extremely distressed, because she was, in fact, all three.

Immediately after the election, anxious students sought safety, at first only among their proven allies and supporters. Some literally barricaded themselves in their living spaces, avoiding classes and other activities out of fear of retaliation. Word spread that this was happening, and in due time it reached the desks of faculty members and administrators. Faculty were particularly incensed and demanded a supportive response from the institution. The Rainbow and their friends constituted not a small proportion of the school's 2,500 students. The plain fact was, not one person wanted to lose any of these students, nor could the school's administrators afford to.

Meetings were called, plans were developed. As it turned out, the simple act of humane caring for students was enormously complex, since communications could easily lead to further targeting of the vulnerable. Informal communication networks among supportive individuals and groups were therefore pressed into service. A wave of texts, emails, and face-to-face meetings followed, each containing information about how and where one might securely find additional services. This included housing accommodations, temporary and emergency financial support, secure transportation, campus safety consultations with law enforcement, buddy systems for walking across campus and sitting with students in class, and counseling and health services, some of which could be offered off site. Counter rallies were organized on campus, with students forming a wall around the targeted groups. The media ran pieces and photos of these events, and at first a backlash was mounted by conservative student groups. But the college president was prepared. Community members were encouraged to avoid events in which violence might be a risk. Police officers were stationed so as to communicate a thorough degree of attention to safety and order. And, perhaps most importantly, the "wall" of support persisted through it all, demonstrating that the campus community would not be intimidated. This took resolve, as the hottest part of the conflict lasted some weeks.

Just as B. F. Skinner taught us, behaviors without reinforcement will extinguish, though at first they may escalate. The whole process takes time. The state's attention, and the governor's, soon turned to other demands, as always happens. The generally hostile climate continued across the region, and this did create a sort of dread and sadness, but the sting had diminished. It's not accurate to say that campus life returned to normal, but its basic functions and missions continued. Targeted students did

> not go away. But it wasn't just they who were engaged and comforted by these events. The entire campus community, faculty, staff, students, and families, admired the courage and resolve of the wee college against much greater forces. Even those who did not necessarily disagree with the governor's platform saw virtue in the school preserving its main purpose: the education of all its students—quiet though they may have been about that.

It is not an accident that education's ancient symbol is the burning oil lamp. IHEs are often in the position of lighting the way, of serving as a beacon of hope and truth, and sometimes this complex role is challenging. An ethic of community responsiveness, another phrase for outreach, is at times the stuff that makes the lamp burn brightly. Heads, and pocketbooks, turn toward that light.

Understanding the Lives of Students

Like outreach, consultations with third parties can address any student thought, feeling, or behavior as it relates to well-being and success. And like outreach, there is virtually no limit to the topics consultations can cover. To provide a glimpse of these topics one need only peer into the lives of students themselves, in their own words. Several years ago, a colleague provided a series of web postings written by college students. The posts, if my memory is correct, were gathered in random fashion from a variety of public internet sources. My memory definitely has failed in one important respect: I can't recall who provided these or exactly when I received them. I apologize for that.

These snippets are simply too good, however, not to record in some way. They provide a glimpse, unsettling at times, into the minds of students. The comments provide us with a sense of what their worlds are really like and therefore some guidance on how we, all of us, might assist them with their needs. They also provide examples of consultative and outreach foci, what it is the community needs to look out for. Spelling and grammatical errors are preserved, as these too are a window into the state of the authors.

Female student

> I've dropped a lot of courses. I've also failed a lot of courses. I don't know my material. I feel like I haven't learned anything. I'm not competent. I've ruined my life. I don't know what I'm going to do. Maybe I will work in fast food for the rest of my life.
>
> I feel like such a loser. I skip final exams. I waste thousands of dollars.
>
> I'm not smart enough. I'm not hard working enough.
>
> I have no future. I can't do anything. I may as well be dead. I'm useless.
>
> My parents should kick me out and leave me homeless. I don't deserve all that they've given me.
>
> I wish I could start over, from the very beginning. I've messed up big time. I've ruined my grades.
>
> I'm getting old. I'm going nowhere. I don't want to face life, it's too scary.
>
> I'll never graduate. Even if I graduate, I'll do nothing with my degree.
>
> I should just die or something. :-(

Male student

> So, I failed my midterm. A huge 45%. The frustrating thing is I know what I'm doing. It's not like I just didn't study,

or not go to class, I did all of that. My prof was even like "What happened?" I didn't do so well on my last quiz, and I'm pretty sure I didn't do well on the one we just had. For awhile now I've been feeling like school is impossible for me. Now, it feels like it is. I don't want to keep going, but I'm afraid of dropping out. I don't konw what to do.

Female student

A couple students including me talked our professior into extending our test date! Heehee! Good for me! I need an extra week!

Female student

i go to university and this is my last semester of classes, or at least, that's the plan, before i do my internship and then one math class in the spring. howveer, my past practice of doing the bare minimum of what's required of me as a student (even less than the bare minimum when it comes to studying for test or reading), has been doing me wrong this semester especially. i have met a guy who has been screwing with my emotions, whether on purpose or not, it doesn't matter i guess. but i am soooo scared that i won't pass some of these classes and then i'll have to stay another semester, here in this wretched town. but i have no energy again. It's like i wish i could be one of those students who can not study and get all a's, but i am not. but although i know my end goal, getting my degree, which as it turns out, again has to be put off till the end of next fall, for other reasons, i cannot seem to focus on that enough to complete my studying, or at least to put more effort into it. i have no job, so it's not time restraints. i don't have a car, so it does take convincing to get myself to walk to campus, if i need to, and i have been skipping more . . . and i don't know . . . does anyone here ever just feel like quitting school, just lie around and do nothing? but then again, that's exacly what i do anyways. i guess i am just here to conplain and ask if anyone else feels like they just do the minimum required of them as students.

Male student

I'm done! My brain is full. It's really sad because the my presentation is less than 2 minutes. What do you do when you just can't stuff anymore in???

Female student

I love school! All the people, the energy, learning, the professors, and everything except the very few parking spaces. LOL I have my first exam in a week, gotta study this weekend. :-)

Female student

I'm soooooooooooooooo nervous! My classes start tomorrow. What if I'm not good enough? What if I fail? What if . . . ? (this coming with someone who has never gotten lower than an A–) uggh. I hate this feeling.

Male student

Classes started up again yesterday. I only have the one class on campus, the other is online. The one class on campus is taught by the same lecturer as the summer math class I just finished. She said we could call her late last week for our grades. She told me I could come by her office and see my final exam, and get my grade.

I haven't done either of those things.

Today I finally emailed her, asking for my grade. She just emailed me back, but I'm too afraid to open it. I know it's going to be awfully close, and I can't stand to see it.

I know, and my T tells me that it's going to be OK to get a B. She says she thinks it would be very good for me to get a B.

I'm too afraid to open the damned email.

I guess it's better than finding out in person, and crying in front of her.

Male student

I woke up yesterday with sore throat, nausea, aches, etc. Still feel yucky.

And I sat down in front of an exam that did not look at all familiar. Not much that looked like anything I had ever seen before. I get depressed when I'm sick anyway, but that just made it that much worse.

I'm pretty sure I won't have an A on the exam. I am currently hoping only that I did well enough to allow me to get an A in the class. I think I can miss 65 or so points, out of 200.

Of course, when I got home again, I could think of how to work out one of the problems. I did get the right answer to that problem, but I had no idea how to set up the equation. {sigh}

I really don't want this to be the time that I find out what happens if I don't get an A. I don't know that I can handle that right now.
Maybe school is too stressful for me.

Female student

I was just diagnosed bipolar ultradian rapid cycling 6 weeks ago, with social phobia 1 week ago, and while I'm getting treatment, none of it is really working yet!! My psychiatrist is confident I'll be ready to go back to school in 5 weeks but I'm soooo scared!! It's like, I don't know if I can handle being in school but if I don't go what do I do? Be a college dropout? Ugh.

As you can see, most of the posts reveal a sense of being overwhelmed by academic demands, some to the point of hopelessness. Another, perhaps more troubling, theme is that few of the students wrote about seeking or asking for help. For this and many other reasons, college mental health services are an absolute necessity for students. Ideally, these services will be well-resourced and thoroughly and repeatedly advertised across campus, in a variety of media. Students tend to dismiss information when they think they will not need it, then suffer from a lack of information when troubles visit them. Institutional support of the mission of college mental health, including consultative support for the entire community, is a vital ingredient in student success, as we see so clearly in the messages provided. Very often, a counselor is the last in a chain of communications concerning student distress. It often spreads outward, from friends, to family, to the resident assistant, to an instructor, and so on. If, at each step of the way, the receiver is well-attuned to mental health issues and resources, the response is more likely to be a competent one. For every increment of competence, the IHE will benefit in increasing probability of retention and academic success.

One could more or less randomly collect narratives from students like the ones presented earlier, or perhaps conduct a series of focus groups to peer behind the curtain into their private lives. Such qualitative research has its place. Large-scale and well-established needs assessments or surveys also have a place, such as that offered by the Center for Collegiate Mental Health, the National College Health Assessment, and the Healthy Minds study. Care must be taken, however, to balance any paradigmatic influences in the instrumentation involved, as was discussed in

Chapter 2. To achieve this, IHEs may incorporate instruments or concepts that consider students from developmental, contextual, or other extrapersonal points of view. An assessment of stress may be undertaken, for example, which will take into account environmental, ecological, or cultural influences on well-being. Perhaps more compelling, an IHE could examine the current state of the languishing vs. flourishing continuum among the student population using instruments designed for that purpose (Diener et al., 2010; Emory University, 2014). Assessments such as these require willingness to honestly and transparently consider any extrapersonal influences on student wellness, but they offer significant probable gains in retention and return on investment. Whether conducted through the counseling service or not, high-quality preventive and consultation work depends entirely on the thoroughness and depth of student needs assessments.

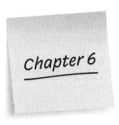

Chapter 6

Paradigm Conflict in Delivering College Mental Health

Given the amount of attention to paradigms and service models provided by most training programs, which is to say very little, it should be no surprise that college mental health professionals cannot know much about conflicts among them—at least at the outset of their careers. After some years of toil, when one begins to discern the ultimate outcomes of policy and funding patterns, and therefore witnesses the impact of same on young adults, one is motivated to learn more, particularly concerning why this is so. All it really takes is working with a client who is directly affected by restricted resources, insurance coverage, and therapeutic interventions that match their circumstances. It is painful to witness the arc of a young person's life being altered or derailed by such things. Today, most people, even the most naive students, have some awareness of the brokenness of health care in the United States, as a result of experiences they have had accessing even the most basic of physical and mental health care. This is particularly true for the latter, in systems that have been wholly subsumed into a strictly medical practice. In that structure, the young adult must navigate the labyrinth of registration, diagnosing, coding, billing, third-party payment, and limitations of service, all of which follow from the economics of the paradigm and model.

Let's start with a few problems that emerge from differences within and between the paradigms. Assuming a strict adherence to any paradigm, which does in fact occur, systems will incorporate their weaknesses into its services, which can then translate into negative outcomes for the client-student. Purely intrapersonal paradigms may ignore the context and growth trajectories of young adults, leading to interventions that make sense in a sterile, content-driven, and academic sense, and may reduce a few symptoms for a while; but clients always regress toward the mean due to the earthly realities of their lives. Extra-personal approaches address negative environments and circum-stances, but, taken to an extreme, overlook the fact of serious mental illness where it may apply. Societal views of clients take them way up river and improve conditions on a grand, popula-tion level, but miss their issues on more interactional, granular, and cellular planes. The spiritual-existential paradigm, as cosmic and transcendent as it may be, can be far afield of the mundane facts and problems of human existence.

Each paradigm has its own strengths and limitations, and that alone is not so much the problem. The problem is stri-dent and strict adherence and the advocacy that goes with it. In mental health, the disciples of a paradigm tend to have the zeal of converts and activists, often due to personal experiences, and sometimes due to economic and status incentives. With this zeal comes enormous energy to affect change, which on the whole is a good thing. Without the tempering that comes with experience and maturity, the disciples demonstrate *paradigmatic blindness*. Such blindness is never a good thing for institutions or their stakeholders, because it will invariably lead to narrow and ineffective responses to need.

Let's further examine the differences, strengths, and limita-tions of the four paradigms so that we can better understand how they may come into conflict.

The *intrapersonal paradigm* addresses the reality of illness and disease through a content-driven rubric that matches interventions—often intrusive—with illness. It offers the prom-ise of rapid reduction in suffering, or at least a degree of man-ageable stasis. While the approach is analytic and rational, in

America it is also costly, owing to the structure of the current health care system. Accessibility is limited. Taken to its logical extreme, the billable encounter may be more relevant than human interaction and therefore get more attention in the workflow, leading to an experience of alienation in users. As noted earlier, this paradigm may overlook the ecological and contextual reality of people and sources of distress. The emerging conflict, then, may be the overvaluing of disease concepts in addressing life problems. Outreach and prevention work in this paradigm tends to focus on mental illness and directing traffic to the intrusive interventions in the most efficient manner possible. In an environment in which cultural or societal psycho-pathogens exist, such efforts produce significant misalignment and confusion in messaging to community members. Illness may be addressed, *but people don't know what else to do*. Further, this may be the prevailing paradigm of health and mental health care in many locations. Changing its direction or focus will, therefore, be difficult and slow.

The *extrapersonal paradigm* speaks to sources of distress in the environment, the community, and circles of human interaction. It works to identify pathogens in those spheres, or negative patterns that result in or aggravate human problems. It is all about the entire context of individuals and groups. Practitioners work with individuals, to help them function more competently in their context, and also with groups and entire communities, to improve their functioning for the greater well-being of all. In this sense, this paradigm affords the possibility of a comprehensive, multilevel, and multiquadrant intervention, and it is compatible with the discipline of community psychology. In short, it may be thorough. A limitation can be lack of attention or discernment concerning illness, especially if the mission translates to siphoning resources away from intrapersonal interventions. Intervening in a community without addressing unconnected symptoms will also be incomplete and unsatisfactory. Consumers may think, *Things are working better, but I still feel bad*.

The *societal paradigm* deals with even broader circles and dynamics. It seeks relief through activism and advocacy for those who are suffering disproportionately. The ills and injustices of an entire society or nation are of interest, as are ways in which these impact individuals, groups, and communities. This paradigm can be the voice of the disenfranchised, the marginalized, the discriminated against, and the abused. Poverty, racism, sexism, and the like are the diagnoses of concern. Alleviating these is believed to trickle down to the level of the individual for his or her benefit. Confronting law, policy, and other institutionalized sources of privilege is a major activity, as is confronting micro-level behaviors that sustain them, such as bystander training focused on sexual assault, harassment, bullying, and racism. This far-reaching paradigm potentially impacts millions, compared to the hundreds or thousands reached by other campus paradigms. Its main limitations involve its slow progress, remoteness of eventual relief in time and space, and sometimes how little good trickles down to individuals. This paradigm is not incompatible with the extrapersonal, and can be seen as an extension of it, so the two can operate well together if that is an intention. Otherwise, community members may sense that *all the noise and advocacy is fine and good, but I am not well and I'm still being victimized.*

The currency of the *spiritual-existential paradigm* is transcendence and wisdom, or seeking the highest and most universal truths, which provide comfort and end suffering. Any faith tradition, or no faith tradition, may be involved. Moral reasoning, ethical behavior, selflessness, and ultimate maturity or actualization may be expected and taught. The paradigm represents the widest, loftiest, and most distant approach to mental health, potentially affecting billions. For these reasons it can also be the slowest and most frustrating because the attitudes and skills involved may take decades to acquire. It also may provide, however, the most thorough and enduring positive change, with some claiming the cessation of all suffering and illness. This is real and very powerful for a great many people. *But it requires the patience of Job*, which unfortunately too few of us possess.

It should be clear how a lack of intentionality in paradigm formation often leads to confusing, contrary, or ineffective responding on campus. Some IHEs exhibit a strict adherence to one paradigm, forsaking all others. Others demonstrate an incoherent mixture of two or more, and may have large, discrepant seams that run between them. Still others may live in an essentially random culture or service model, which might change from day to day. Such conflicts emerge through the efforts of a rogue, errant, or abusive administrator, or a singular focus on economics, or capitulation to guild politics, or outright laziness, or by thoughtless default.

Developing Systems by Default

Every once in a blue moon, you will learn of a psychologist, counselor, or social worker who dwells in the upper adminisphere of higher education. Perhaps this is more common among smaller IHEs. Otherwise, it is usual for this group to consist of career administrators and those with business and financial acumen. In today's climate of shrinking state dollars, this is not totally unwise. Former college deans and, not uncommonly, physicians by training are also represented. Their attention is naturally drawn to operations that have greater financial impact, in both expenditure and revenue. The notion of "too big to fail" may come into play. And, compared to other student services units on campus, which often include health care, this reflects similar patterns and pressures at the national level. When upper-level administrators are gathered around the boardroom table, then, deliberating over funding priorities, it can be tempting to privilege such systems without respect to long-term consequences for campus culture and well-being. In this way, the intrapersonal paradigm, particularly of the medical variety, often becomes the default student-response system. In terms of finances, it is not hard to see why this is so. Further, the guild of medicine actively lobbies accordingly. And even further, since mental health professionals themselves are often unaware of paradigmatic issues, administrators may be underinformed about the internecine politics of mental health.

Here is an example. Some years ago, the AMA launched its Scope of Practice Partnership (SOPP, American Medical Association, 2018), which, in its essence, seeks to legislatively protect the practice of medicine against what it sees as an effort among nonphysician health-care professionals "to expand their scope of practice." Buried in the details of SOPP is also an effort to place all allied health care under the supervision of medicine, in state statutes, licensing boards, and of course in practices. Other mental health professionals were not pleased by this development. Attaining independent licensure has been a major battle for mental health professionals—for psychologists dating back to the 1950s. The SOPP initiative smelled of economic motives, as physicians saw their revenue being negatively impacted in the current health care system—which it is, along with everything and everyone else in a system that is widely recognized as being broken.

About the same time that the SOPP was developed, the notion of integrated health care appeared more frequently, and I think for the same reasons, though it was cloaked in language of superior patient safety and outcomes, as well as cost savings, which had not been clearly demonstrated at the time. Since then there is equivocal evidence to support the idea (Flanagan, Damery, & Combes, 2017; Balasubramanian et al., 2017). On its surface, it is logical to conclude that benefits may accrue mainly for those in rural areas and those who are less able to advocate for themselves, such as the very young, the very old, and the incompetent, since these groups may find it more challenging to articulate and advocate for their own needs. However, the Kaiser Permanente Health System, considered a model of health-care integration, has not been able to demonstrate significant cost savings (Pho, 2013). Furthermore, in a National Demonstration Project designed to coach 36 practices in setting up an integrated Patient Centered Home Model, it was "found that there wasn't much difference in outcomes whether the practice was coached or not, and there was practically no difference in quality (5% change in mostly meaningless metrics) and no difference in costs or patient experience in these practices over 26 months of follow up" (Young, 2018). The movement spread to higher education, which has seen a limited but painful increase in medical and mental health mergers, and not without strife and loss.

Young adults, however, are capable of directing their own affairs, and college provides a perfect opportunity for them to learn how to do this in every sphere of their lives; it would be decidedly contrary to the mission of higher education to strip emerging adults of autonomy in learning how to be effective advocates for their own health care. Further, concerns about the negative impact on the delivery of psychotherapy within a medical model have been outlined (Elkins, 2009). Among the most salient problems Elkins noted in such settings is an obscuring of psychotherapy as an interpersonal process when viewing it as a medical intervention for mental illness. This is a significant conceptual problem for college students specifically, as many of them access therapy services for support, skill development, and personal growth, making the therapeutic relationship or alliance a critical feature in this form of help.

You can't blame people for their advocacy. This is a permanent part of the human condition, it seems, and has likely been so for millennia. But we are living in an era in which questions of privilege and social justice are frequently raised, and for good reason. Because we are a more educated and better-resourced population than were our ancestors, we can and should be more circumspect and less reflexive in establishing our educational priorities. This theme is embedded deeply in the national politics of the United States and other countries. In the case of counseling centers, being more circumspect means taking into account all aspects of human diversity, all alternatives for the enhancement of human welfare, and all points of view and paradigms that alleviate human suffering. In short, it is possible for us to be comprehensive in college mental health. Is it challenging and difficult to do so? You bet. But it is possible, and for that reason alone we ought to try. To repeat: a guiding question for everyone ought to be, What is the nature of my community, and what orientations will serve it best?

The Realities of Mergers with Medical Departments

Integration has become a buzzword of sorts, and like all buzzwords, its meaning is never unambiguously clear. It is not even clear what the word means in higher education mental health. To start, a plethora of seemingly interchangeable terms are being used to describe this pattern of structure: *integration, merger, colocation, collaboration, holistic services, one-stop shopping, conjoint services*, and more. In addition, since offices at all IHEs are relatively "nearby," even on large campuses, one could argue that IHEs already offer convenience and heightened communicative collaboration. In fact, unless you live in an unusual town, you will never see such convenient or low-cost health care once you leave college.

Data from recent Association for University and College Counseling Center Directors (AUCCCD) surveys, previously cited, show that approximately 15% of member centers report some sort of combined structure, be it purely administrative or, at the other extreme, purely physical. Even more compelling, 68% of these leaders do not agree on the precise nature of the arrangement. This last data point strongly suggests that the effort to combine services was not done in a clear and rational manner, one easily understood by managers. If this is so, it follows that any consideration of paradigm and service model was likely cursory or nonexistent. What, then, was the point of combining services? In the absence of any obvious answer, stakeholders may assume that the reason was money, the saving or the making of it. Other more subterranean motives, which actually do sometimes trump profit, such as bad-faith decisions about constructing services, are not likely to be known by the center's staff members or even its direct managers. Even a profit motive is often an illusion; there may be savings in the short-term budgeting sense, but long-term or hidden costs may wash out or surpass the revenue lines. Finally, given that college counseling center directors report that 94.9% of center clients do not need coordination of care by medical providers aside from psychiatry (AUCCCD, 2017), astute observers will be mystified by claims to the contrary.

Brunner, Wallace, Keyes, and Polychronis (2017) also expose at least two flaws in the merger logic in addition to definitional problems. This logic places mergers, and specifically the comprehensive counseling center model, in opposition to one another, when in reality the structures each offer something unique and could even coexist on the same campus. In fact, they already have, for decades. Brunner et al. also identify the loss of a center's developmental mission, citing individuals, groups, and communities as a worrisome fallout of mergers—particularly, I believe, in thoughtless, hostile, or forced integrations. Here, the center faces a harmful extraction from "the fabric of campus life," which is dangerous for all the reasons already covered in previous chapters. Put simply, the IHE faces the loss of future growth and development through broad and competent consultative work performed by trained college mental health professionals. Such a loss is incalculable.

There are other, perhaps more pernicious potential losses, especially in settings that adhere to an intrapersonal paradigm and medical service model. These include a loss of heterogeneity in professional culture or organizational structure and work processes. When the compass is set on as strict a course as this combination can sometimes dictate, the work culture can fail to recognize diversity in all its dimensions. A loss of diversity in thought and orientation toward humans will result in a *loss in the multiplicity and complexity of points of view of students*. It bears repeating that students may be viewed through a wide variety of lenses and dimensions; developmental, contextual, ecological, feminist, social justice, occupational, human service, public health, biological, spiritual, and other dimensions all have something significant to offer in the alleviation of human suffering. When a service has an incomplete and narrow focus, it will have incomplete and narrow outcomes. It is also worth emphasizing that such losses can occur without any intention whatsoever.

Losses in point of view have tremendous implications at all levels of IHE functioning. In mental health services that have been reduced to the clinical role, students may be seen as biological organisms or bags of health behaviors. The campus community and its members may be seen as part of the intervention delivery system, their role being to get students into the delivery system. Prevention-oriented services may be limited or nonexistent and may focus only on the public health orientation to human problems. Quick, on-the-fly consultations with a faculty member who is concerned about a student are not of interest. Organizational development within the IHE isn't even on the radar. This is all to say that multidimensional, multilayered, complex, and systems-oriented approaches vanish or fail to thrive. In theory, strict adherence to any paradigm and model can result in accompanying losses, as described in the sections on paradigm limitations. So why do these paragraphs focus on medical mergers? There is only one reason: in my entire career I have never heard or read about large-scale efforts by any *other* paradigm to subsume the others. This makes that particular type of integration a major potential stumbling block, about which all practitioners and higher education professionals need to be informed.

What Can We Realistically Deliver?

By now you may be asking, With all the choices and points of view involved, aren't we at risk of assembling an incoherent, Frankensteinian mental health system on campus? This is a fair question. Is an IHE honestly able to address a fuller range of needs and perspectives? Some argue that IHEs have morphed into an Amazon-style customer service corporate culture, along with the readoption of standing in loco parentis, when it had no business doing so. I have heard more than one administrator wish he or she could dismantle services and programs with a "full-service" or "high-touch" orientation, I suppose because of the many real headaches involved. But alas, the consumer has come to expect them in return for the tuition dollar. Nonetheless, and putting that aside, can we really provide a full service? With all our hearts, minds, and motives in the right place, I believe we can. And therefore we should try.

But providing a full service does involve making important choices. In an ideal IHE world, with unlimited resources, administrators would be able to develop a seamless range of services representing different points within each of the four paradigms. (Some well-endowed schools actually come pretty close to this.) Such an approach could theoretically address a wide array of needs and encompass diverse points of view. Also ideal would be laying out the framework ahead of time, much as a progressive city planner might do, in order to reduce the likelihood of incoherency or redundancy. For most schools this is rarely possible; but it is always possible to improve upon what we offer. In the world of limited resources, which is to say the world in which most of us live, we can critically examine what we are providing from a paradigmatic point of view. It is crucial this not be done in a checkbox fashion, in which we say, "Oh, XYZ sort of does that, let's plug that in here." Rather, it is the spirit of the paradigm from which we work. It is also essential that this work not be derailed by economic or political points of view. While the financial aspects of service models are not irrelevant, they cannot be the sole compass by which we navigate. When these are privileged, student needs or issues will surely go unaddressed.

In this way we map out what we are currently doing, thereby determining points in the paradigms that are unoccupied. In these gaps we can then identify points at which we can most easily address a need or perspective (the low-hanging fruit). We can also identify needs or perspectives that are critical in our community (the musts and shoulds). Since we are limited, we cannot develop something for every conceivable point in the paradigms, and it may not even be necessary to do so. What we are looking for here is the *best possible coverage* of needs and perspectives in our community, given the state of its resources, and working from the paradigmatic point of view. We are looking to cover the spectrum implied by the paradigms.

Conclusion: A Road Map for Success

Paradigms and service models are the templates, the motifs, by which we construct mental health services. For the most part, neither IHE administrators nor college counseling professionals receive much training about these templates. For this reason such services are often constructed in a problematic manner, or one in which prevailing orientations hold sway, which results in needs and perspectives being lost or unfilled. These factors may also be responsible for conflicts within and between services and the professionals who staff them. Dynamics that occur in mergers, especially of the thoughtless variety, are often rife with conceptual and paradigmatic confusion, which in turn siphons off precious energy better suited for comprehensively resolving student needs. In this book I seek to provide a framework for conceptualizing paradigms and the service models that flow from them, and in so doing to fill an educational gap for IHEs. I also seek to provide a method or process of identifying community needs based on paradigms and, more importantly, subsequently meeting those needs.

The paradigms fall along a spectrum. This spectrum charts the human journey, from deep within persons, to the immediate environment around them, to the society in which they live, and beyond, to the metaphysical and transcendental aspects of existence. Each paradigm occupies a meaningful and valuable place on the spectrum because each offers unique solutions to human needs. Within each paradigm there are other spectra, which represent the extreme end points of the paradigm and everything in between. These spectra within a spectrum offer full and diverse points of view of students and their needs, thus offering suggestions as to what services and programs are best, and most realistically, suited to the community (fig. 3).

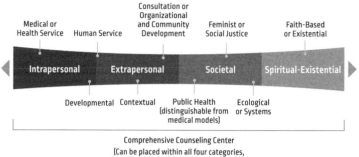

Figure 3. College Mental Health Paradigm Spectrum

We are not obliged to cover every conceivable point in the spectrum, and it would not be financially possible to do so anyway. But an IHE should ask itself what points are possible and desirable to capture for their particular campus. Community culture and needs ought to drive this search. Start with an assessment of existing programs, services, and models. Locate them on the paradigm spectrum. Include any assessment data being collected concerning their outcomes and effectiveness. This is an opportunity for the IHE to determine the viability of its programs and their relation to community goals, culture, and needs. Redundancies may be reduced, and ineffective or incongruent programs eliminated. What remains may be viewed as the framework upon which new approaches can be constructed and existing ones enhanced or reformulated. Let me offer a few guiding questions:

- What are the issues (problems, concerns, behaviors, etc.) on our campus that can be seen as predominantly originating from within individuals?
  - What approaches to these issues have we not implemented? What do we currently do that needs improvement? What do we do well?

- What are the issues that can be seen as predominantly originating from between individuals, groups, and communities?
  - What are the negative contexts that our students face? What contexts promote learning, health, and well-being?

- What are the issues that can be seen as predominantly originating from between and among entire societies or cultures?
  - What groups are at odds with each other? What policies, laws, and customs sustain or perpetuate conflict and dis-order? What is needed to promote peace and justice?

- What are the issues that can be seen as predominantly originating from the state of being human, of life itself and its meaning created by humans?
  - What does our community do that promotes self-actualization, mature interdependence and altruism, and transcendence of challenges in life?

After developing a sense of the paradigm or paradigms of interest, attention must turn to developing the service model for the college counseling center. Service models are not to be confused with service structures, although too often this is what occurs. A service structure is merely an organizational chart; it is two-dimensional and communicates little to nothing about direction. A model will be multidimensional and encompass philosophy, vision, and mission, as well as strategic goals and objectives and the components and services that are intentionally designed to achieve them. It communicates a course the IHE will take in the delivery of counseling services. To an extent, paradigms offer a sense of philosophy, vision, and direction. Ultimately though, the IHE will need to define targets for student and community growth. The targets will be hallmarks of ideal or maximum development (see fig. 4) and what is theoretical but captured by keywords. For students, Chickering's vectors of student development provide excellent keywords, but these may be derived from other theoretical points of view.

Chickering's vectors:

- Developing competence
- Managing emotions
- Moving through autonomy toward interdependence
- Developing mature interpersonal relationships
- Establishing identity
- Developing purpose
- Developing integrity

The arc of development provides a perspective that goes well beyond the college years. It is helpful to consider the lifelong impact that education—or any other service, for that matter—will have on youth. Anyone can be on a path that leads to the actualization of an "ideal" self, and anyone may stray off that path, or "off the arc." But the nice part is that we can, at any time, return to that path or return to the arc. College is one vital time during which such questions and formulations are highly relevant, and college counseling services are one important vehicle for this work.

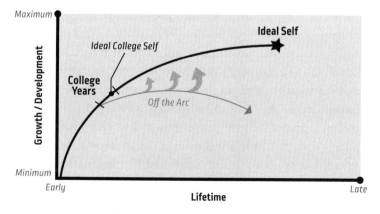

Figure 4. Arc of Student Development

Communities, the context in which students live, are also in need of development, a target, and keywords to describe the target. Examples may include:

- Financial support
- Employment opportunities
- Safety
- Clean and sustainable environment
- Stability

- Inclusion
- Green and gathering spaces
- Political representation
- Neighborliness
- Cooperation
- Interdependence

Who does the work of defining paradigm, model, and targets? Administrators and financial wizards should absolutely be involved in providing answers, but they alone will not be able to address the questions satisfactorily. The group doing this work must also include psychologists, sociologists, anthropologists, clergy, philosophers, artists, poets and writers, change makers and peacemakers, ethicists, community leaders, physicians and nurses, and many more. It is serious business, and it requires serious effort and not a small amount of time and other resources. The task is to lay down the DNA of a humane, supportive, and just community, one that assists the largest number possible in their learning and creation of a healthy future.

Gather the leaders. After identifying the group, set aside at least three days for deliberations. One week would be better. Choose an independent facilitator to guide the meetings, someone who can be impartial but will follow the basic structure outlined here. Meet off campus in a location conducive to reflection, creativity, and healthy, vigorous interaction. Ask the president to announce the objective in unambiguous terms, perhaps something like: "We are here to create our response and care systems from the ground up, without regard to personal or disciplinary agenda, and without any tethering to what we have done in the past." Develop a set of ground rules ahead of the meeting. These should include (1) all participants having an equal opportunity to speak and provide perspectives, (2) discussions being oriented toward addressing the stated questions, and (3) any agendas and needs being clearly identified at the beginning of the meeting. There may be other ground rules specific to a particular IHE, as long as these are not inconsistent with the stated objective.

Present student and campus data. No act of creation can be successful or sustainable if it does not incorporate an honest look at known facts and an admission of what is not known. Start by collecting data on the questions outlined in previous chapters, presented again here.

- What is known about the prevalence of diagnosed mental illness, including substance abuse and addiction, in the community? Are some disorders more frequent than others? In whom? What is the state and range of campus and local medical health services? What is the state and range of campus and local counseling and psychotherapy resources? What is the state of health insurance in the area? Do all practitioners understand, respect, and work within each other's professional cultures and values?

- What are the most common physiological stresses for students and others? What is the state of housing, food supply and deserts, clothing needs for the climate, safety and exposure or vulnerability to crime? What are the most common criminal offenses, and who are the most frequent victims? Where can one go to get help about everything in this list?

- Describe the "psychological ecosystem" of the area. Identify the major components in this system. In what areas might one feel unwelcome or threatened? In what areas might one find affiliation and support? How difficult is it to get there and to gather? How easy or difficult is it to belong?

- What is the prevailing social, religious, and political climate of the area? Who are the privileged? Who are the disenfranchised or marginalized? Who or what is assisting the

latter? Does the institution provide or connect to these resources?

- Who works in the intersections of diverse groups? Who are
the joiners, and the peacemakers? Who are the dividers,
the splitters, the separators? How quickly can the people
find or avoid these groups? What is the state of spiritual
and ethics resources in the community?

- What opportunities do the people have to increase esteem
in self and others? How can they safely explore, create, express, and manifest or actualize their identities and gifts?
With whom and where would this happen? Would anything
or anyone interfere with these growth processes?

- What key laws, regulations, and policies provide for or
constrict the well-being of the people? Is the institution
involved in advocating for enhancements or corrections of
these issues?

Determine the expectations for outcome. The group must make
choices about what it will provide to its community beyond the
degrees it awards students and the services it offers them. In
many ways, this set of questions may encompass aspects of the
IHE's brand, but it should not be limited to that. Sometimes a
brand may actually be a source of student and community problems, especially if it has been applied in a rigid, impossible-to-
achieve manner. Participants must be able to take a step back
and candidly examine what the IHE actually provides in terms
of implicit or felt experience. The list may be long and may contain sensitive or, to some, unsavory items, like those we covered
earlier:

- Status or image
- Avoiding stigma
- Employment
- Income
- A meaningful life
- Social connections
- Return on investment
- Social justice

- Preserving privilege
- Good grades
- Fidelity to family and their beliefs
- Contentment with career
- Clear pathways to advancement
- Entertainment
- Amenities and comforts

- Minimal disruption
- Challenge
- Support for development
- Teaching independence
- Teaching civic responsibility
- Marketable skills
- Life skills
- Safety
- Adventure

At this point the group will need to determine which items need enhancing and which need minimizing or eliminating, at least from a point of view of *emphasis*. Once this has been determined, the group will have addressed three very large questions: who are we, who do we want to be, and where do we want to go? The desire is to be extremely thorough in the search for these answers, as this sets the stage for the next steps.

Present the paradigm, service model, and spectrum templates. This part of the meeting will include a description and an explanation of the material. Since most graduates of the helping professions have not been exposed to these concepts, there is likely to be a good deal of cognitive dissonance involved. Allow time for questions and discussion, and for the incorporation of new schema in their minds, but remember the objective of the meeting. To create new response and care systems one must have a starting point, an orientation or map by which to navigate. These templates provide the broadest, most inclusive mapping available, in my opinion. These are as good a place to start as any, and it is important to champion them and to draw any wanderers back to why they are there. There may be some time for reflecting about how well or poorly the current array of services fit into these templates, but again the idea is to start from scratch, so this rehearsal must be limited.

Make choices about the ideal template spots on which to focus. At this stage the group should still be dreaming. Resist the temptation to quickly move into practicalities. That will come later. It will be necessary to have an understanding of how current services fit in, but recall that participants need to address the issues and problems identified in previous steps. The guiding questions here are: What points on the paradigms and its spectra and what service models will ideally address our community needs? Also, what are the top five to 10 needs or priorities? The key word here is *ideal*. Dream a lot and dream big. The answers provided at this point may well form a very long-term strategy, applicable for decades to come. Though the focus in this book has been college mental health, the framework may apply to many other services or programs if questions about origins of human problems are relevant to them.

Determine what is fiscally possible. Participants will need some notion of the IHE's budgetary health, of what is currently allocated and what could be reallocated. Without this information the exercise will be akin to shooting in the dark. But it is not just about the now; the group should determine the priorities as established in preceding stages and focus on what could be and how they can get there. This will include discussions about funding strategies and campaigns to raise any needed monies.

Set specific goals for funding, advancing toward the priorities, and moving beyond them. These are the practicalities, and people often get bogged down in them. While initial goals are important, the most crucial aspect of the process is to create and follow a dream for many years. Participants will need to develop, say, two-year, five-year, and 10-year plans. For this reason a project director should be named and tasked with follow-up and convening the planning group periodically for a review of progress and recommended adjustments. The ultimate goal is implementing the broadest, most comprehensive set of services possible, occupying the ideal locations within the paradigms, and creating the service models that best fit the intended plan to address the identified community needs.

The field of higher educations has for a long time needed a rubric, or template, for the rational construction of helping communities and mental health services. Without it, services and programs may be erected willy-nilly and be subject to ephemeral forces having to do with politics, guild issues, the funding of the health-care environment, or a rogue and charismatic administrator. The needs of today's college student are far too complex to be adequately addressed by trends that come and go, and a tremendous amount of time has been wasted on orienting services around such trends. For the template to be useful it must also incorporate philosophical views of humans and the problems they face. I wrote this book in an attempt to address this gap.

Colleges and universities are literally fighting over the admission of students. In order to attract and retain them, IHEs must develop services that match the diversity of students and the campus cultures in which they live. The return on investment does not occur when a student is invited, welcomed, even treated something like royalty, but then experiences a failure to live up to the promise. Time and money is well spent when a great deal of preparation goes into the creation of a community that truly addresses the full range of student attributes and needs.

I urge campus leaders to consider as background the paradigms, service models, and road map for bringing it all to fruition presented here. I strongly believe in the absolute necessity of alternatives and giving each one full consideration as one evaluates one's community. At the same time, this process should never stifle creativity. The template provided here is loose enough to cobble together the elements, even new elements not yet known, in a meaningful way for any college campus. I hope you and others find this helpful in your efforts to intentionally and ethically address student needs.

References

Al-Debei, M. M., El-Haddadeh, R., & Avison, D. (2008, August). *Defining the business model in the new world of digital business*. Proceedings of the Americas Conference on Information Systems, Toronto, Canada.

American College Health Association. (2006). *National College Health Assessment: Spring 2006 reference group executive summary*. Hanover, MD: Author.

American College Health Association. (2007). *National College Health Assessment: Fall 2007 reference group executive summary*. Hanover, MD: Author.

American College Health Association. (2010). *National College Health Assessment: Fall 2010 reference group executive summary*. Hanover, MD: Author.

American College Health Association. (2016). *National College Health Assessment: Fall 2016 reference group executive summary*. Hanover, MD: Author.

American Medical Association. (2018). *Scope of practice partnership*. Retrieved from https://www.ama-assn.org/about/scope-practice #Scope of Practice Partnership.

American Psychiatric Association. (2013). *Diagnostic and statistical manual of mental disorders* (5th ed.). Washington, DC: Author.

American Psychological Association. (2017). *Ethical principles of psychologists and code of conduct*. Washington, DC: Author.

American Psychological Association. (2017). *Stress in America: The state of our nation*. Retrieved from http://www.apa.org/news/press /releases/stress/index.aspx.

American University and College Counseling Center Directors. (2015). *Directors survey monograph*. Indianapolis, IN: Author.

American University and College Counseling Center Directors. (2016). *Directors survey monograph*. Indianapolis, IN: Author.

American University and College Counseling Center Directors. (2017). *Directors survey monograph*. Indianapolis, IN: Author.

Archer, J., & Cooper, S. (1998). *Counseling and mental health services on campus: A handbook of contemporary practices and challenges*. Hoboken, NJ: Jossey-Bass.

Balasubramanian, B. A., Cohen, D. J., Jetelina, K. K., Dickinson, L. M., Davis, M., Gunn, R., . . . Green, L. A. (2017). Outcomes of integrated behavioral health with primary care. *Journal of the American Board of Family Medicine, 30*(2), 130–139.

BBC News. (2018, June 25). University student suicide rates revealed. Retrieved from https://www.bbc.com/news/health-44583922.

Blidner, R. (2015, March 17). MIT cuts back on course loads after 2 students commit suicide in same week. *New York Daily News.* Retrieved from http://www.nydailynews.com/news/national /mit-lightens-load-2-student-suicides-1-week-article-1.2152311.

Brunner, J., Wallace, D., Keyes, L. N., & Polychronis, P. D. (2017). The comprehensive counseling center model. *Journal of College Student Psychotherapy, 31*(4), 297–305.

Brunner, J. L., Wallace, D. L., Reymann, L. S., Sellers J., & McCabe, A. G. (2014). College counseling today: Contemporary students and how counseling centers meet their needs. *Journal of College Student Psychotherapy, 28*(4), 257–324.

Budinger, M. C., Drazdowski, T. K., & Ginsburg, G. S. (2013). Anxiety-promoting parenting behaviors: A comparison of anxious parents with and without social anxiety disorder. *Child Psychiatry & Human Development, 44*(3), 412–418.

Burlingame, G. M., & Fuhriman, A. (1987). Conceptualizing short-term treatment: A comparative review. *Counseling Psychologist, 15*(4), 557–595.

CBS News. (2018, June 7). Dramatic rise in suicides is "more than a mental health issue," CDC says. Retrieved from https://www .cbsnews.com/news/suicide-rates-rise-more-than-a-mental-health -issue-cdc-says/?ftag=CNM-00-10aag7e.

Center for Collegiate Mental Health. (2016). *Annual report.* University Park, PA: Author.

Center for Collegiate Mental Health. (2017). *Annual report.* University Park, PA: Author.

Centers for Disease Control and Prevention. (2015). *Age-adjusted death rates for selected causes of death, by sex, race, and Hispanic origin: United States, selected years, 1950–2014* [Table 17]. Atlanta, GA: Author.

Centers for Disease Control and Prevention. (2015). *Death rates for suicide, by sex, race, Hispanic origin, and age: United States, selected years, 1950–2014* [Table 30]. Atlanta, GA: Author.

Centers for Disease Control and Prevention. (2015). *Serious psychological distress in the past 30 days among adults aged 18 and over, by*

selected characteristics: United States, average annual, selected years,
1997–1998 through 2013–2014 [Table 46]. Atlanta, GA: Author.

Centers for Disease Control and Prevention. (2018, June). *VitalSigns:*
Suicide. Atlanta, GA: Author.

Chickering, A. W., & Reisser, L. (1993*). Education and identity.* (2nd ed.).
San Francisco, CA: Jossey-Bass.

Conkin, P. K. (2000). *A requiem for the American village.* Lanham, MD:
Rowman & Littlefield.

Cosgrove, L. (2010). *Diagnosing conflict-of-interest disorder.* AAUP.
Retrieved from https://www.aaup.org/article/diagnosing-conflict
-interest-disorder#.WpFI0OhKvrc.

Costa, K. L. (2016). Could unlearning help our college mental health
crisis? *HuffPost.* Retrieved from https://www.huffingtonpost.com
/kristen-lee-costa/could-unlearning-help-our_b_9464188.html.

Costello, T. (2016). Hacking of health care records skyrockets. *NBC*
News. Retrieved from https://www.nbcnews.com/news/us-news
/hacking-health-care-records-skyrockets-n517686.

Cottone, R. R. (1992). *Theories and paradigms of counseling and psycho-*
therapy. Needham Heights, MA: Allyn & Bacon.

Cottone, R. R. (2007). Paradigms of counseling and psychotherapy,
revisited: Is social constructivism a paradigm? *Journal of Mental*
Health Counseling, 29(3), 189–203.

Cummings, N. A., & Sayama, M. K. (1995). *Focused psychotherapy:*
A casebook of brief, intermittent psychotherapy throughout the life cycle.
London: Psychology Press.

Davenport, R. (2017). The integration of health and counseling services
on college campuses: Is there a risk in maintaining student patients'
privacy? *Journal of College Student Psychotherapy, 31*(4), 268–280.

Diener, E., Wirtz, D., Tov, W., Kim-Prieto, C., Choi, D., Oishi, S., &
Biswas-Diener, R. (2010). New well-being measures: Short scales
to assess flourishing and positive and negative feelings. *Social Indi-*
cators Research 97(2), 143–156.

Doward, J. (2013). Psychiatrists under fire in mental health battle. *The*
Guardian. Retrieved from https://www.theguardian.com/society
/2013/may/12/psychiatrists-under-fire-mental-health.

Duncan, B. L., & Miller, S. D. (2000). *The heroic client: Doing client-*
directed, outcome-informed therapy. San Francisco, CA: Jossey-Bass.

Eiser, A. (2011). The crisis on campus. *Monitor on Psychology, 42*(8), 18.

Elkins, D. N. (2009). The medical model in psychotherapy: Its limitations and failures. *Journal of Humanistic Psychology, 49*(1), 66–84.

Ellwood, P. M. (2005). Models for organizing health services and implications of legislative proposals. *Milbank Quarterly, 83*(4).

Emory University. (2014). *Overview of the mental health continuum short form (MHC-SF)*. Atlanta, GA: Emory University.

Falco, M. (2012). Early therapy can change brains of kids with autism. CNN. Retrieved from https://www.cnn.com/2012/10/31/health/autism-therapy-brain/index.html.

Flanagan, S., Damery, S., & Combes, G. (2017). The effectiveness of integrated care interventions in improving patient quality of life (QoL) for patients with chronic conditions: An overview of the systematic review evidence. *Health and Quality of Life Outcomes, 15*, 188.

Frances, A. J. (2012). Psychiatric mislabeling is bad for your mental health. *Psychology Today*. Retrieved from https://www.psychologytoday.com/blog/dsm5-in-distress/201205/psychiatric-mislabeling-is-bad-your-mental-health.

Garvey, J. C. (Ed.). (2014). *Theory to practice: Translating the process of student development at the University of Alabama*. Tuscaloosa, AL: Author.

Glass, G. S., & Tabatsky, D. (2014). *The overparenting epidemic: Why helicopter parenting is bad for your kids, and dangerous for you too!* New York, NY: Skyhorse.

Greenberg, R. P. (2016). The rebirth of psychosocial importance in a drug-filled world. *American Psychologist, 71*(8), 781–791.

Hansen, J. T. (2007). Should counseling be considered a health care profession? Critical thoughts on the transition to a health care ideology. *Journal of Counseling and Development, 85*(3), 286–293.

Hayes, S. C., Villatte, M., Levin, M., & Hildebrandt, M. (2011). Open, aware, and active: Contextual approaches as an emerging trend in the behavioral and cognitive therapies. *Annual Review of Clinical Psychology, 7*, 141–168.

Headley, J. (2013). *It's not about the nail* [Video]. YouTube. Retrieved from https://www.youtube.com/watch?v=-4EDhdAHrOg.

Healthy Minds Network. (2018). Web information retrieved from http://healthymindsnetwork.org/.

Huey, S. (2016). Challenging a mandate to adopt electronic health records (EHRs). *National Psychologist*. Retrieved from http://nationalpsychologist.com/2016/05/challenging-a-mandate-to-adopt-electronic-health-records-ehrs/103277.html.

Insurance Journal. (2018). 13 South Carolina hospital employees fired in 2017 over privacy breaches. Retrieved from https://www.insurance journal.com/news/southeast/2018/03/02/482185.htm.

International Association for Counseling Services. (2016). *Standards for university and college counseling services.* Alexandria, VA: Author.

Jed Foundation. (2017). Students with mental troubles on rise; colleges add suicide response teams, counselors. Retrieved from https:// www.jedfoundation.org/students-with-mental-troubles-on-rise/.

Jed Foundation. (2018). Jed Consultation Services. Retrieved from https://www.jedfoundation.org/jed-consultation-services/.

Kalia, M. (2002). Assessing the economic impact of stress—the modern day hidden epidemic. *Metabolism, 51*(6 Suppl 1), 49–53.

Keyes, C. L. (2002). The mental health continuum: From languishing to flourishing in life. *Journal of Health and Social Behavior, 43*(20), 207–222.

Kuhn, T. S. (1970). *The structure of scientific revolutions* (2nd ed.). Chicago, IL: University of Chicago Press.

Laska, K. M., Gurman, A. S., & Wampold, B. E. (2014). Expanding the lens of evidence-based practice in psychotherapy: A common factors perspective. *Psychotherapy, 51*, 467–481.

Lewis, J. M., Beavers, W. R., Gossett, J. T., & Phillips, V. A. (1989). *No single thread: Psychological health in family systems.* New York, NY: Brunner/Mazel.

Lichstein, K. L. (2017). Insomnia identity. *Behaviour Research and Therapy, 97*, 230–241.

Merikangas, K. R., Nakamura, E. F., & Kessler, R. C. (2009). Epidemiology of mental disorders in children and adolescents. *Dialogues in Clinical Neuroscience, 11*(1), 7–20.

Morrill, W. H., Oetting, E. R., & Hurst, J. C. (1974). Dimensions of counselor functioning. *Journal of Counseling and Development, 52*(6), 354–359.

National Alliance on Mental Illness. (2012). *College students speak: A survey report on mental health.* Arlington, VA: Author.

National Association of Social Workers. (2017). *Code of ethics of the National Association of Social Workers.* Washington, DC: Author.

Patten, S. B., Wang, J. L., Williams, J. V., Currie, S., Beck, C. A., Maxwell, C. J., & el-Guebaly, N. (2006). Descriptive epidemiology of major depression in Canada. *Canadian Journal of Psychiatry, 51*, 84–90.

Patterson, T. (2016). Why do so many graduate students quit? *The Atlantic*. Retrieved from https://www.theatlantic.com/education /archive/2016/07/why-do-so-many-graduate-students-quit /490094/.

Pho, K. (2013). Health reform faces tension with integrated health systems [Blog post]. *KevinMD.com*. Retrieved from https://www .kevinmd.com/blog/2013/04/health-reform-faces-tension -integrated-health-systems.html.

Physicians for a National Health Program. (n.d.). *Health care systems— four basic models*. PNHP. Retrieved from http://www.pnhp.org /single_payer_resources/health_care_systems_four_basic_models .php.

Piper, E. (2017). This is not a day care. It's a university! [Blog post]. Retrieved from https://www.okwu.edu/blog/2015/11/this-is-not -a-day-care-its-a-university/.

Polychronis, P. D. (2018). Integrated care, shared electronic records, and the psychology profession: A cautionary tale for counseling centers. *Journal of College Student Psychotherapy*. doi:10.1080/87568225. 2018.1489745.

Post, R. M., Snyder, B. M., Byer, M. L., & Hurowitz, G. (n.d.). What's my M3? Retrieved from https://whatsmym3.com/.

Public Broadcasting System. (2011). Steve Jobs—one last thing. Re- trieved from http://www.pbs.org/show/steve-jobs-one-last-thing/.

Sampath, R. (2017). The myth of the coddled college student. *HuffPost*. Retrieved from https://www.huffingtonpost.com/rini-sampath /the-myth-of-the-coddled-c_b_8760620.html.

Schulman, M. (2012). Five ethical choices you will have to make in college. *USA Today*. Retrieved from http://college.usatoday.com /2012/08/22/5-ethical-choices-you-will-have-to-make-in-college/.

Schwartz, A. (2011). Rate, relative risk, and method of suicide by students at 4-year colleges and universities in the United States, 2004–2005 through 2008–2009. *Suicide and Life-Threatening Behavior, 41*(4), 353–371.

Schwartz, B. (2003). *The paradox of choice: Why more is less*. New York, NY: HarperCollins.

Screening for Mental Health. (2018). [Web information]. Retrieved from www.mentalhealthscreening.org.

Siegel, D. J. (2014). *Brainstorm: The power and purpose of the teenage brain*. London: Penguin.

Steegmuller, F. (Ed. and Trans.) (1982). *The letters of Gustave Flaubert, 1857–1880.* Cambridge, MA: Harvard University Press.

Thomas, J. (2014). Caution flags raised over ACA electronic records requirement. *National Psychologist.* Retrieved from http://national psychologist.com/2014/09/caution-flags-raised-over-aca-electronic -records-requirement/102621.html.

Thombs, B. D., Coyne, J. C., Cuijpers, P., de Jonge, P., Gilbody, S., Ioannidis, J. P., . . . Ziegelstein, R. C. (2012). Rethinking recommendations for screening for depression in primary care. *Canadian Medical Association Journal, 184*(4), 413–418.

Tough, P. (2013). *How children succeed: Grit, curiosity, and the hidden power of character.* New York, NY: Random House.

Twenge, J. M. (2000). The age of anxiety? Birth cohort change in anxiety and neuroticism, 1952–1993. *Journal of Personality and Social Psychology, 79*(6), 1007–1021.

Twenge, J. M., Joiner, T. E., Rogers, M. L., & Martin, G. N. (2017). Increases in depressive symptoms, suicide-related outcomes, and suicide rates among U.S. adolescents after 2010 and links to increased new media screen time. *Clinical Psychological Science, 6*(1), 3–17.

Wampold, B. E., & Imel, Z. E. (2015). *The great psychotherapy debate.* New York: Routledge/Taylor-Francis.

Wickelgren, I. (2012). Trouble at the heart of psychiatry's revised rule book. *Scientific American.* Retrieved from https://blogs.scientific american.com/streams-of-consciousness/trouble-at-the-heart-of -psychiatrys-revised-rulebook/.

World Health Organization. (1992). *International statistical classification of diseases and related health problems* (10th ed.). Geneva, Switzerland: Author.

World Health Organization. (2018). Public health, environmental and social determinants of health. Retrieved from http://www.who.int /phe/about_us/en/.

World Health Organization. (2018). Social determinants of health. Retrieved from http://www.who.int/social_determinants/sdh _definition/en/.

Young, R. (2018). The tiny gains of patient-centered medical homes. Are they worth it? [Blog post]. *KevinMD.com.* Retrieved from https://www.kevinmd.com/blog/2018/03/tiny-gains-patient -centered-medical-homes-worth.html.

Index